Chemotherapy

International Journal of Experimental and Clinical Chemotherapy
Founded 1959 as 'Chemotherapia'

KARGER

Printed in Switzerland on acid-free paper by Reinhardt Druck, Basel

Appears bimonthly: 1 volume per year (6 issues)

Guidelines for Authors

Chemotherapy

Submission

Only original papers written in English are considered and should be sent to:

Dr. H. Schönfeld
S. Karger AG
Editorial Office Chemotherapy
P.O. Box
CH–4009 Basel (Switzerland)
Tel. +41 61 306 1357
Fax +41 61 306 1434
E-Mail l.haas@karger.ch

Mailing address for courier deliveries only:

Allschwilerstr. 10
CH–4055 Basel (Switzerland)

Manuscripts should be submitted in duplicate (with two sets of illustrations of which one is an original), typewritten double-spaced on one side of the paper, with a wide margin. The final version of your manuscript and illustrations should also be submitted on disk. For details refer to 'Disk Submission' or www.karger.com/journals/disksub.htm. Editorial review and copy-editing will be executed from the disk version of your manuscript.

Conditions

All manuscripts are subject to editorial review. Manuscripts are received with the explicit understanding that they are not under simultaneous consideration by any other publication. Submission of an article for publication implies the transfer of the copyright from the author to the publisher upon acceptance. Accepted papers become the permanent property of 'Chemotherapy' and may not be reproduced by any means, in whole or in part, without the written consent of the publisher. It is the author's responsibility to obtain permission to reproduce illustrations, tables, etc. from other publications.

Arrangement

Title page: The first page of each paper should indicate the title, the authors' names, and the institute where the work was conducted. A short title for use as running head as well as the full address of the author to whom correspondence should be sent are also required.

Full address: The exact postal address complete with postal code must be given at the bottom of the title page. Please also supply phone and fax numbers, as well as your e-mail address.

Key words: For indexing purposes, a list of 3–10 key words in English is essential.

Abstract: **Each paper needs an abstract of up to 150 words structured with subheadings as follows: Background, Methods, Results, Conclusion(s).**

Small type: Paragraphs which can or must be set in smaller type (case histories, test methods, etc.) should be indicated with a 'p' (petit) in the margin on the left-hand side.

Footnotes: Avoid footnotes. When essential, they are numbered consecutively and typed at the foot of the appropriate page.

Tables and illustrations: Tables and illustrations (both numbered in Arabic numerals) should be prepared on separate sheets. Tables require a heading and figures a legend, also prepared on a separate sheet. For the reproduction of illustrations, only good drawings and original photographs can be accepted; negatives or photocopies cannot be used. Due to technical reasons, figures with a screen background should not be submitted. When possible, group several illustrations on one block for reproduction (max. size 144 × 196 mm) or provide crop marks. On the back of each illustration, indicate its number, the author's name, and 'top' with a soft pencil.

Color illustrations: Up to 6 color illustrations per page can be integrated within the text at the reduced price of CHF 660.– / USD 545.00 per page. Color illustrations are reproduced at the author's expense.

References: In the text identify references by Arabic numerals [in square brackets]. Material submitted for publication but not yet accepted should be noted as 'unpublished data' and not be included in the reference list. The list of references should include only those publications which are cited in the text. Do not alphabetize; number references in the order in which they are first mentioned in the text. The surnames of the authors followed by initials should be given. There should be no punctuation other than a comma to separate the authors. Cite all authors, 'et al,' is not sufficient. Abbreviate journal names according to the Index Medicus system. (Also see International Committee of Medical Journal Editors: Uniform requirements for manuscripts submitted to biomedical journals. N Engl J Med 1997;336:309–315.)

Examples

(a) Papers published in periodicals: Sun J, Koto H, Chung KF: Interaction of ozone and allergen challenges on bronchial responsiveness and inflammation in sensitised guinea pigs. Int Arch Allergy Immunol 1997;112:191–195.

(b) Monographs: Matthews DE, Farewell VT: Using and Understanding Medical Statistics, ed 3, revised. Basel, Karger, 1996.

(c) Edited books: Parren PWHI, Burton DR: Antibodies against HIV-1 from phage display libraries: Mapping of an immune response and progress towards antiviral immunotherapy; in Capra JD (ed): Antibody Engineering. Chem Immunol. Basel, Karger, 1997, vol 65, pp 18–56.

(d) Papers published in electronic format: Black CA: Delayed type hypersensitivity: Current theories with a historic perspective. Dermatol Online J 1999;5:7.
http://dermatology.cdlib.org/DOJvol5num1.

Page charges

There is no page charge for papers of 6 or fewer printed pages (including tables, illustrations and references). Each additional complete or partial page is charged to the author at CHF 275.– / USD 196.00. The allotted size of a paper is equal to approx. 12 manuscript pages (including tables, illustrations and references).

Galley proofs

Unless indicated otherwise, galley proofs are sent to the first-named author and should be returned with the least possible delay. Alterations made in galley proofs, other than the correction of printer's errors, are charged to the author. No page proofs are supplied.

Reprints

Order forms and a price list are sent with the galley proofs. Orders submitted after the issue is printed are subject to considerably higher prices.

KARGER

Fax +41 61 306 12 34
E-Mail karger@karger.ch
www.karger.com

The Guidelines for Authors are available at:
www.karger.com/journals/che/che_gl.htm

Chemotherapy

General Information

Publication data: 'Chemotherapy' is published 6 times a year. Volume 47 with 6 issues appears in 2001.

Subscription rates: Subscriptions run for a full calendar year. Prices are given per volume.
Personal subscription:
Subscription + postage and handling
CHF 376.– + CHF 27.40 Europe
CHF 376.– + CHF 40.80 Overseas
USD 289.00 + USD 27.40
+ online subscription per volume:
CHF 39.–/USD 30.00
(Must be in the name of, billed to, and paid by an individual. Order must be marked 'personal subscription'.)
Institutional subscription:
Subscription + postage and handling
CHF 752.– + CHF 34.20 Europe
CHF 752.– + CHF 51.– Overseas
USD 578.00 + USD 34.20
+ online subscription per volume:
CHF 58.–/USD 45.00
Airmail postage: CHF 36.–, USD 30.00.
(Extra per volume.)

Microforms: Please direct all enquiries and orders to: University Microfilms Inc.
300 North Zeeb Road, P.O. Box 1346
Ann Arbor, MI 48106-1346 (USA)

Advertising: Correspondence and rate requests should be addressed to the Publisher.

Subscription orders: Orders can be placed at agencies, bookstores, directly with the
Publisher S. Karger AG, P.O. Box,
CH–4009 Basel (Switzerland)
or with any of the following distributors:
Deutschland: S. Karger GmbH, Postfach
D–79095 Freiburg
France: Librairie Luginbühl
36, bd de Latour-Maubourg
F–75007 Paris
Great Britain, Ireland: S. Karger Publishers
58 Grove Hill Road
Tunbridge Wells, Kent TN1 1SP, UK
USA: S. Karger Publishers, Inc.
26 West Avon Road, P.O. Box 529
Farmington, CT 06085, USA
India, Bangladesh, Sri Lanka:
Panther Publishers Private Ltd.
39, 6th Cross
Wilson Gardens
Bangalore 560 027, India
Japan: Katakura Libri, Inc.
2F, Marushima Bldg, 4-6-17, Yushima,
Bunkyo-ku, Tokyo 113-0034, Japan

Change of address: Both old and new address should be sent to the subscription source.

Single issues: Information can be obtained through the Publisher.

Bibliographic indices: This journal is regularly listed in bibliographic services, including *Current Contents®*.

Book Reviews: Books are accepted for review by special agreement.

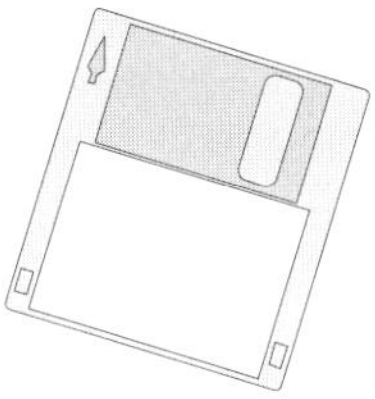

Disk Submission

A **comprehensive version** of these guidelines for the **submission of manuscripts and illustrations on disk** can be accessed online under **www.karger.com/journals/disksub.htm** or requested as a leaflet from the editorial department.

Please follow the general rules on style and arrangement in the **'Guidelines for Authors'** of the journal. Submit a **double-spaced printout** of your manuscript matching the file on disk exactly.

Technical Information

Store only data pertinent to this manuscript. Include your fonts (screen and printer fonts for Macintosh).
For a **text only** manuscript, use a 3.5-inch disk. For **text and illustrations,** use 3.5 or 5.25 Magneto Optical Disc; CD-ROM (DOS or hybrid); iomage Zip/DOS (100 MB), or 44 MB, 88 MB or 200 MB SyQuest. Compress extensive data using ZIP format.

Data Description

Label your disk with the **title of the journal or book** for which it is submitted; a **short version** of the paper's title; your **name,** postal and e-mail address, fax and phone number; **hard and software** used, including the version; and the **complete list of the file names.** File names consist of eight characters before the dot identifying the file and three characters after the dot identifying the application.

Text and Format

The **preferred word-processing package is MS-Word.** Other commonly used PC text programs and ASCII formats are accepted.
Update your data when you revise subsequent to the reviewer's or editor's decision and mark revisions clearly. Manuscripts accepted for publication are subject to **copy editing:** changes and/or questions will be marked in the manuscript, which will be returned to you with your disk and the galley proofs for checking.
Enter your text continuously flush left. Do not use any layout functions. Do not split words at the end of a line. **Do not use indentations.** Use a blank line before and a hard return at the end of paragraphs. **Arrange headings flush left.** Insert only **one space after punctuation marks.** Insert Greek letters, mathematical symbols etc. with your word-processing program. Use **boldface and italics** as well as sub- and superscript where appropriate. **Tables are part of the text** and should be placed at the end of the text file. Separate the individual parts of a table by lines. Use the tabulator instead of spaces. Format operation data on one line in the same column. **Legends to illustrations are part of the text** and should also be listed at the end of the text file.

Illustrations

Store illustrations as separate files: do not integrate them in your text. Export **line drawings/vector graphics** as TIF, EPS or WMF format. Use Photoshop for processing and retouching **scanned half-tone images.** Save the original scan and the processed version. Export **black and white or color images** as TIF or EPS format in their anticipated size in print.
For detailed information on how to submit illustration data on disk please consult the leaflet or **www.karger.com/journals/disksub.htm.**

KARGER

Fax +41 61 306 12 34
E-Mail karger@karger.ch
www.karger.com

The Journal Home Page is available at:
www.karger.com/journals/che

KI 98 DISK

A thorough discussion of biological, diagnostic and clinical aspects

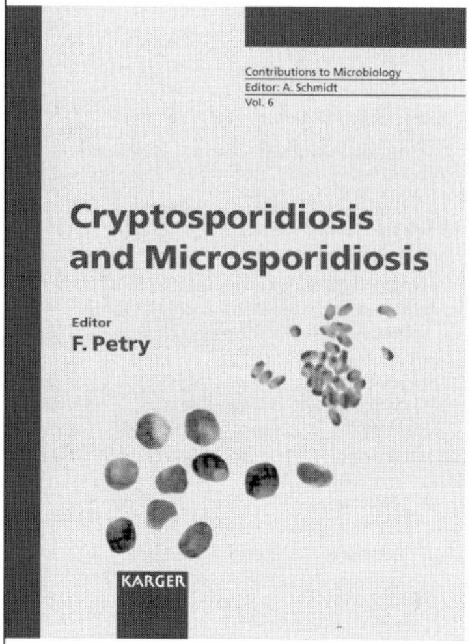

Cryptosporidiosis and Microsporidiosis

Editor
Franz Petry

Microbiology; Infectious Diseases; Parasitology; Gastro-enterology; AIDS; Immunosuppression; Tropical Medicine

Cryptosporidia and microsporidia are protozoan parasites that have emerged as human pathogens over the last two decades. With the coming of AIDS they have been recognised as important opportunistic pathogens of patients with an impaired host defence system. For both groups of pathogens, chemotherapeutic intervention is extremely limited. To date, cryptosporidiosis and microsporidiosis are severe and life-threatening opportunistic infections in AIDS patients and cryptosporidiosis is a major cause of diarrhea in infants and children in developing countries.
This volume provides a comprehensive overview of the biology of the pathogens as well as the diagnosis and clinical aspects of the diseases they cause. The host immune responses against *Cryptosporidium* and the immunology of human microsporidiosis are reviewed in detail. Further topics discussed include the epidemiology and strain variation of *Cryptosporidium parvum*, the epidemiology and zoonotic aspects of microsporidia, and gene discovery in *Cryptosporidium*. Offering a well-written and very comprehensive description of what is currently known about these emerging pathogens, this book is a valuable reference for clinical microbiologists and specialists in infectious diseases, epidemiologists in the public health sector, and physicians in general and internal medicine.

Contents

KI 00247

www.karger.com/bookseries/comii

Contributions to Microbiology, Vol. 6
Series Editor: Schmidt, A. (Wuppertal)
ISSN 1420–9519

Cryptosporidiosis and Microsporidiosis
Editor: Petry, F. (Mainz)
XII + 268 p., 28 fig., 9 in color, 19 tab.,
hard cover, 2000
CHF 218.– / DEM 283.– / USD 189.25
Prices subject to change
DEM price for Germany, USD price for USA only
ISBN 3–8055–7050–3

KARGER

Order Form

Please send: ____ copy/ies

Postage and handling free with prepayment

Payment:
☐ Check enclosed ☐ Please bill me

Please charge to my credit card
☐ American Express ☐ Diners ☐ Eurocard
☐ MasterCard ☐ Visa

Card No.: ____________

Exp. date: ____________

Orders may be placed with any bookshop, subscription agency, directly with the publisher or through a Karger distributor.

Fax to: +41 61 306 12 34
S. Karger AG, P.O. Box, CH–4009 Basel (Switzerland)
E-Mail orders@karger.ch, **www.karger.com**

Name/Address: ____________

Date: ____________

Signature: ____________

Chemotherapy

Quinolones Are Not All the Same: Different Safety Profiles for Specific Compounds

Proceedings of the Roundtable Discussion Held in Conjunction with the 10th European Congress of Clinical Microbiology and Infectious Diseases

Stockholm, Sweden, May 30, 2000

Guest Editor
Ethan Rubinstein, Tel Aviv, Israel

7 figures and 25 tables, 2001

KARGER

Basel · Freiburg · Paris · London · New York ·
New Delhi · Bangkok · Singapore · Tokyo · Sydney

The current Meeting and Publication were made possible by an educational grant from Daiichi Pharmaceutical Co., Ltd.

Editorial Development by
BIOMEDIS International Ltd.

S. Karger
Medical and Scientific Publishers
Basel · Freiburg · Paris · London
New York · New Delhi · Bangkok
Singapore · Tokyo · Sydney

Drug Dosage
The authors and the publisher have exerted every effort to ensure that drug selection and dosage set forth in this text are in accord with current recommendations and practice at the time of publication. However, in view of ongoing research, changes in government regulations, and the constant flow of information relating to drug therapy and drug reactions, the reader is urged to check the package insert for each drug for any change in indications and dosage and for added warnings and precautions. This is particularly important when the recommended agent is a new and/or infrequently employed drug.

P.O. Box, CH–4009 Basel (Switzerland)
Printed in Switzerland on acid-free paper by
Reinhardt Druck, Basel
ISBN 3–8055–7322–7

KARGER

Fax+ 41 61 306 12 34
E-Mail karger@karger.ch
www.karger.com

Vol. 47, Suppl. 3, 2001

Chemotherapy

Contents

KARGER

Fax+41 61 306 12 34
E-Mail karger@karger.ch
www.karger.com

Access to full text and tables of contents, including tentative ones for forthcoming issues:
www.karger.com/journals/che/che_bk.htm

Chemotherapy

Chemotherapy 2001;47(suppl 3):1–2

Introduction

Ethan Rubinstein, Symposium Chairperson

Department of Internal Medicine and Unit of Infectious Diseases,
Tel Aviv University School of Medicine, Tel Aviv, Israel

Fluoroquinolones now stand as one of the most significant classes of antimicrobials, being the most commonly prescribed oral antibiotics in the US. The earliest agents in this class were beneficial in many clinical situations and were very well tolerated. This led to a rapid rise in interest in these compounds, and a corresponding development of newer agents with greater efficacy. Over the past few years, there have been a number of new fluoroquinolones developed, and some now marketed globally. Interest in such development has led to the emphasis on research into structure–activity relationships to help develop increasingly effective compounds. This has resulted in newer agents having greater potency, a broader spectrum of activity, and greater activity against resistant organisms. They maintain long half-lives, which in turn has allowed for once-daily administration. These improved features have been associated with the rise of fluoroquinolones as a class, making them the first choice in many infectious diseases in place of cephalosporins, macrolides, and older agents.

Along with this increase in activity, changes in side-effect profiles have been reported. Previously, it was believed that the fluoroquinolones were relatively similar in terms of their incidence and spectrum of adverse events. However, recent reports have highlighted substantial differences among agents concerning side-effect profiles, and this has led to interest in clarifying their structure–side effect relationships. By gaining a greater understanding of the roles that specific substitutions attached to the quinolone nucleus have, the possibility is there for safer drugs to be developed and unsafe ones withdrawn before market exposure. Thus, no longer can the fluoroquinolones be considered interchangeable. The clinician is now able to choose agents that are both effective and well tolerated.

To bring together all the strands of data detailing the structure–activity and structure–side effect relationships, a special roundtable discussion was chaired by the author of this introduction, Professor Ethan Rubinstein, Tel Aviv University School of Medicine, Israel. The discussion participants were experts from

KARGER

Fax + 41 61 306 12 34
E-Mail karger@karger.ch
www.karger.com

0009–3157/01/0479–0001$17.50/0

Accessible online at:
www.karger.com/journals/che

Ethan Rubinstein, MD
Department of Internal Medicine and Unit of Infectious Diseases
Chaim Sheba Medical Center, Tel Aviv University School of Medicine
Tel-Hashomer, 52621 Israel
Tel. +972 3 530350, Fax +972 3 5347081, E-Mail unit@netvision.net.il

around the world, who were able to clarify the differences among the fluoroquinolones based upon safety and tolerability issues. The papers following this introduction report on each individual presentation, as well as the informative discussion that was held at the end of the session. The first paper, by the present author, will set the scene for the reader, with a clear summary of the structure–activity and structure–side effect profiles of individual fluoroquinolones. Professor Claude Carbon, Bichat-Claude Bernard Hospital, Paris, France, then clarifies differences among individual fluoroquinolones, describing the relative incidences of specific adverse events. Professor Jacques F. Acar, Fondation Hôpital Saint-Joseph, Paris, France, will compare fluoroquinolones to other commonly used agents, such as macrolides and β-lactams, before describing the ecological impact of different antimicrobials upon the normal human gastrointestinal flora. With the possibility that such changes in flora may relate to the propensity of different agents to cause resistance, this is one area that needs to be fully addressed. By gaining a greater understanding of which agents are likely to be associated with the development of future resistance, the clinician will be able to prescribe safer drugs. Adding to the preclinical data will be the presentation by Professor Hartmut Lode, City Hospital Berlin-H-Heckshorn, Berlin, Germany, who looks at the differences in pharmacological features among the fluoroquinolones. These features are responsible for different profiles of the fluoroquinolones in terms of their bioavailability, penetration, and drug–drug interactions. With many patients taking more than one drug, it is important for interactions to be documented, and for the effect of individual agents to be analysed. This will allow for the use of agents that are less likely to interact with other commonly used medications, thereby ensuring greater safety and more effective drugs.

Clinical data following extensive use of levofloxacin will then be presented to assess the safety and efficacy of fluoroquinolones, with particular emphasis upon levofloxacin. This will be assessed first from a US perspective, with results presented by Dr. James B. Kahn, Ortho-McNeil Pharmaceutical, Inc., N.J., USA, reporting on the latest clinical trial data, surveillance studies, and spontaneous reports. These incidence rates will be compared to results from Japan, as reported by Dr. Katsuro Yagawa, Daiichi Pharmaceutical Co., Ltd., Tokyo, Japan, who will provide a comprehensive analysis of levofloxacin safety using Japanese and world-wide data from over 130 million prescriptions.

This roundtable discussion was developed with the aim of helping the clinician decide which antimicrobial to use. It is now well recognised that efficacy cannot be the sole criterion, but must be balanced against other factors, including safety, tolerability, cost, and administration options. The question as to which is the best agent to use can be a difficult one to answer, and one that has engendered a great deal of debate in the past. The roundtable discussion brings together experts who have distinguished and long careers in the field of infectious disease. They will help to develop a consensus differentiating the individual fluoroquinolones based upon evidence gained throughout the world, using both preclinical and clinical data.

Chemotherapy

Chemotherapy 2001;47(suppl 3):3–8

History of Quinolones and Their Side Effects

Ethan Rubinstein

Department of Internal Medicine and Unit of Infectious Diseases, Tel Aviv University School of Medicine, Tel Aviv, Israel

Key Words

Fluoroquinolones · Adverse drug reactions · Adverse events · Safety · Structure–activity relationships · Structure–side-effect relationships

Abstract

Fluoroquinolone development from 1985 to the present was reviewed. Severe drug adverse events were noted for enoxacin, pefloxacin and fleroxacin, which were phototoxic. Temafloxacin was associated with severe hemolytic–uremic syndrome, lomefloxacin caused phototoxicity and central nervous system (CNS) effects, and sparfloxacin was associated with phototoxicity and QTc prolongation. Tosufloxacin caused severe thrombocytopenia and nephritis, and hepatotoxicity was reported for trovafloxacin. Grepafloxacin was withdrawn due to cardiovascular effects, and clinafloxacin was associated with phototoxicity and hypoglycaemia. The structure of the quinolones directly relates to both their activity and side-effect profiles. The relationship among specific substituents attached to the quinolone nucleus are clarified. The incidence of specific adverse events associated with individual fluoroquinolones was reviewed in a five-year post-marketing surveillance (PMS) study in Japan, in which a total adverse drug reaction (ADR) rate of 1.3% was found for levofloxacin, compared to total ADR rates of 3.3% for pazufloxacin, 3.6% for tosufloxacin, 4.5% for gatifloxacin and 5.4% for balofloxacin. Gastrointestinal effects were the most common adverse events for all fluoroquinolones. Levofloxacin had the lowest rate of CNS effects and skin adverse events among the agents listed.

Introduction

After reviewing the history of the development of fluoroquinolones, one may be left with the impression that this is a class of antimicrobials strewn with discarded agents,

KARGER

Fax + 41 61 306 12 34
E-Mail karger@karger.ch
www.karger.com

© 2001 S. Karger AG, Basel
0009–3157/01/0479–0003$17.50/0

Accessible online at:
www.karger.com/journals/che

Ethan Rubinstein
Department of Internal Medicine and Unit of Infectious Diseases
Chaim Sheba Medical Center, Tel Aviv University School of Medicine
Tel-Hashomer, 52621 (Israel)
Tel. +972 3 530350, Fax +972 3 347081, E-Mail unit@netvision.net.il

Table 1. Toxicity of selected fluoroquinolones

Agent	Year	Side effect
Enoxacin	1985	Severe drug interactions
Pefloxacin	1985	Phototoxicity, tendinitis, etc.
Fleroxacin[a]	1990	Phototoxicity, CNS effects
Temafloxacin[a]	1992	Haemolytic–uremic syndrome (92 cases)
Lomefloxacin	1993	Phototoxicity, CNS effects
BAY y 3118[b]	1993	Phototoxicity
Sparfloxacin	1994	Phototoxicity, QTc prolongation
Tosufloxacin[b]	1996	Severe thrombocytopenia, nephritis
Trovafloxacin[a]	1999	Hepatotoxicity (140 cases)
Grepafloxacin[a]	1999	Severe cardiovascular events
Clinafloxacin[b]	1999	Phototoxicity, hypoglycaemia

[a] Withdrawn in Europe.
[b] Clinical development stopped.
Modified from reference 3.

left by the wayside as unacceptable side effects became apparent. However, that would be taking a simplistic view. While some agents have not stood the test of time, others, notably ofloxacin, ciprofloxacin, and now levofloxacin, have proven their safety following extensive use around the world. Thus, a comprehensive review of fluoroquinolone development should also note these extremely successful compounds before looking at the ones that have not proven reliable. The fluoroquinolones can be divided into safe and non-safe compounds according to the generation. Norfloxacin, a first-generation compound, has proven to be relatively non-toxic. Ofloxacin and ciprofloxacin, both second-generation agents, are safe and well tolerated. Levofloxacin, a third-generation compound, has an excellent safety profile [1]. Currently, there is insufficient evidence regarding levofloxacin to confirm the safety of moxifloxacin, a fourth-generation fluoroquinolone, but it does appear safe at present [2].

The toxicity of selected fluoroquinolones has been recognised since 1985 (table 1) [3]. In 1985, severe drug interactions associated with the cytochrome P450 system were noted for enoxacin, and in the same year, pefloxacin was reported to be phototoxic and to cause tendinitis. In 1990, fleroxacin was reported to cause phototoxicity as well as central nervous system (CNS) effects [4], leading to its withdrawal. In 1992, 95 cases of severe haemolytic–uremic syndrome were associated with temafloxacin [5]. Since then, a number of compounds have been noted to cause severe adverse drug reactions (ADRs). Lomefloxacin has been associated with phototoxicity and CNS effects, sparfloxacin with phototoxicity and QT interval prolongation, and tosufloxacin with severe thrombocytopenia and nephritis. In 1999, trovafloxacin had to be withdrawn due to 140 cases of hepatotoxicity, and grepafloxacin was withdrawn due to cardiovascular effects, mainly QT interval prolongation, and due to taste perversion. The latest casualty has been clinafloxacin, which is associated with phototoxicity and severe hypoglycaemia. This list of failed fluoroquinolones focuses attention on the need to distinguish among individual agents so as to identify which are safe and well tolerated.

Clarifying Fluoroquinolone Structure–Activity Relationships

The structure of quinolones is directly related not only to their activity, but also to their side-effect profiles. Thus, there has been heightened interest in clarifying the structure–activity and structure–side-effect relationships of the fluoroquinolones [6]. The structure of all clinically important fluoroquinolones is based upon the modified dual-ring system (fig. 1). The basic molecule can be either a quinolone nucleus with a nitrogen in position 1, or a naphthyridone nucleus, which has an extra nitrogen in position 8 and a carboxyl group attached to position 3. The nitrogen at position 1 cannot be replaced, although different groups can be attached at this position. The majority of compounds have an oxygen attached at position 4 and a fluorine at position 6 for both of these basic molecules. All of the other positions are capable of having different constituents. Each of the positions around the rings is associated with specific activities, such as potency, Gram-positive activity, gyrase binding, and pharmacodynamic effects. Thus, the antibacterial activity of fluoroquinolones depends not only on the quinolone or naphthyridone nucleus, but also on the substituents attached at the nucleus periphery. These substituents exert their effect by adding to the affinity for bacterial enzymes, thereby changing cell pharmacokinetics or bioavailability.

Elucidation of these structure–activity relationships has revealed the following: Position 1 is associated with potency and pharmacokinetic attributes of individual agents, while position 2 is involved in gyrase binding. The third carboxyl and fourth carbonyl groups are essential for antibacterial activity because of their action in gyrase binding and bacterial transport. Position 5 controls potency and Gram-positive activity, and the activity increases in the following order:

$OH < F < Cl < OCH_3 < NH < CH_3$

The fluorine at position 6 controls gyrase binding and potency. Position 7 is involved in potency, antibacterial spectrum, and pharmacokinetics, and C-7 substituents may interact with bacterial enzymes, and may be involved in controlling the permeability into bacterial cells. Position 8 is associated with pharmacokinetic features and activity against anaerobic bacteria.

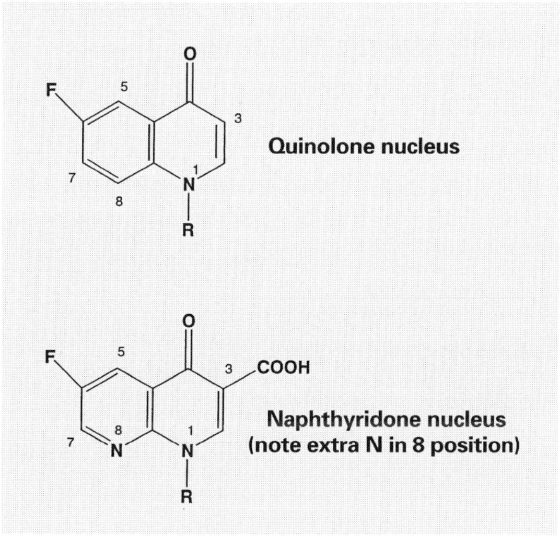

Fig. 1. The basic molecules.

Structure–Side Effect Relationships Reviewed

In the same way as there are specific fluoroquinolone structure–activity relationships, it has been recognised that certain side effects

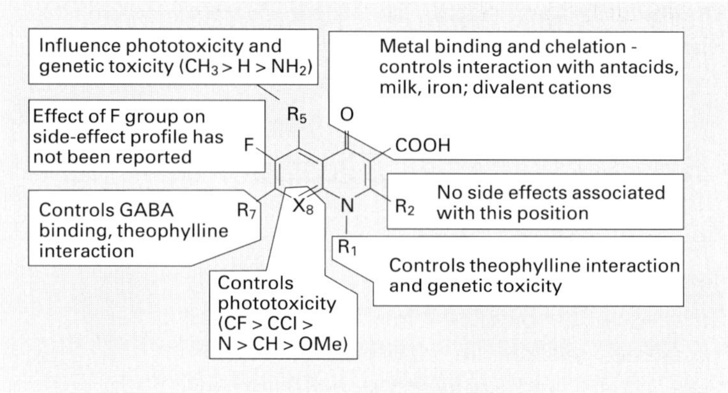

Fig. 2. Quinolone structure–side-effect relationships. Modified from reference 6.

are associated with constituents at specific sites around the quinolone nucleus (fig. 2) [6]. Research has shown that position 1 controls theophylline interaction and genetic toxicity. There is no known side effect associated with position 2. The oxygen at position 3 and the carboxyl at position 4 are both involved in chelation and metal binding, and thus they interact with antacids, milk, iron, and other divalent cations such as Mg^{++} or Ca^{++}. Position 5 is important in influencing phototoxicity and genetic toxicity. In this position, a methyl group causes more adverse events than a hydrogen, while an amino compound in this position is the least likely to cause these problems.

No effect has been noted for the fluorine at position 6. Position 7 controls γ-aminobuytric acid (GABA) binding activity in the brain and is therefore responsible for some CNS side effects. In addition, it is also involved in theophylline interaction. Position 8 is important in terms of structure–adverse event relationships. It has been shown to be the major position mediating phototoxicity, and a fluorine in this position has stronger phototoxic potential than chlorine or nitrogen.

Further elucidation of these structure–side effect relationships has revealed that dihalogenated quinolones are associated with a high degree of phototoxicity. Identified quinolones include lomefloxacin and sparfloxacin, as well as clinafloxacin, for which the development has recently been discontinued due to this side effect.

Fluoroquinolones with a naphthyridone base, and an additional third nitrogen, have been associated with considerable phototoxicity. One example of such a compound is enoxacin, which has a high potential for phototoxicity and can interact with theophylline. Tosufloxacin is associated with similar problems, as is trovafloxacin. One of the concerns regarding new drugs is the potential for gemifloxacin to be associated with high rates of phototoxicity. While there have been no clinical indications of this to date, gemifloxacin does contain the naphthyridone base, which is strongly implicated in these reactions.

Hepatotoxicity has not been associated with the naphthyridone structure itself, but it does appear that the presence of two or three nitrogens is associated with this problem. While temafloxacin does not have a naphthyridone structure, the nitrogen in the ring is similar to trovafloxacin, which is strongly associated with hepatotoxicity.

Table 2. Overall incidence of adverse events of fluoroquinolones: US and European data

Fluoroquinolone	Total AE (%)	GI (%)	CNS (%)	Skin (%)
Ciprofloxacin	5.8	3.4	1.1	0.7
Ofloxacin	4.2	2.6	0.89	0.53
Levofloxacin	2–9.9	5.1	0.2–1.1	0.2
Sparfloxacin	13.7–25.3[a]	11.4	4.2	5.1
Grepafloxacin	47.0[a]	15	5	2.0

[a] Drug-related incidence.
AE = adverse event, GI = gastrointestinal, CNS = central nervous system.
Adapted from reference 3.

Table 3. Incidence of adverse events of new fluoroquinolones: Japanese data

Fluoroquinolone	Total AE (%)	GI (%)	CNS (%)	Skin (%)
Pazufloxacin[a]	3.3	2.1	0.7	0.4
Tosufloxacin[a]	3.6	2.3	0.75	0.4
Levofloxacin[b]	1.3	0.52	0.10	0.10
Gatifloxacin[a]	4.55	2.85	0.7	0.8
Balofloxacin[a]	5.4	2.6	1.0	0.85

[a] Adapted from reference 3.
[b] Adapted from five-year PMS data on levofloxacin in Japan, Daiichi Pharmaceutical Co., Ltd., Tokyo, Japan.
AE = adverse event, GI = gastrointestinal, CNS = central nervous system.

Safety of Levofloxacin

The large number of modifications made to the chemical structure of individual fluoroquinolones have resulted in a wide range in the incidence of ADRs. The overall incidence of adverse events associated with their use in the US and Europe reveals levofloxacin to be the safest among this group, with a total adverse event rate of only 2.4%. This is in contrast to sparfloxacin with a total adverse event rate of 13.7–25.3%, and a high rate of 47% for grepafloxacin. Even ofloxacin and ciprofloxacin, both very well tolerated agents, are associated with a greater number of ADRs than levofloxacin. The main ADRs with levofloxacin are gastrointestinal, occurring in 5.1% of patients, and it has a very low rate of phototoxicity (0.2%), CNS (0.2–1.1%), and other ADRs compared to other agents (table 2) [3].

Data from Japan provides further evidence supporting the excellent safety profile of levofloxacin. The total drug-related adverse event rate for levofloxacin in Japan was 1.3%, the lowest among the other new fluoroquinolones tested. Pazufloxacin had a rate of 3.3%, tosufloxacin 3.6%, gatifloxacin 4.55% and balofloxacin 5.4%. Gastrointestinal effects were the most common for all fluoroquinolones, but while the other four agents all had rates of over 2%, the rate of gastrointestinal effects associated with levofloxacin was much lower at 0.52% (table 3) [3]. Levofloxacin also had the lowest rates of CNS and skin adverse events among the agents listed. The safety of levofloxacin has been confirmed by US, European, and Japanese data. All findings have demonstrated the excellent tolerability of levofloxacin, showing it to have a lower rate of adverse events compared to the new and older fluoroquinolones presently available.

References

1 Langtry HD, Lamb HM: Levofloxacin. Its use in infections of the respiratory tract, skin, soft tissues and urinary tract. Drugs 1998;56:487–515.

2 Lipskey BA, Baker CA: Fluoroquinolone toxicity profiles: A review focusing on newer agents. Clin Infect Dis 1999;28:352–364.

3 Ball P, Mandell L, Niki Y, Tillotson G: Comparative tolerability of newer fluoroquinolone antibacterials. Drug Saf 1999;21:407–-421.

4 Bowie WR, Willetts V, Jewesson PJ: Adverse reactions in a dose-ranging study with a new long-acting fluoroquinolone, fleroxacin. Antimicrob Agents Chemother 1989;33:1778–1782.

5 Blum MD, Graham DJ, McCloskey CA: Temafloxacin syndrome: review of 95 cases. Clin Infect Dis 1994;18:946–950.

6 Domagala JM: Structure-activity and structure-side-effect relationships for the quinolone antibacterials. J Antimicrob Chemother 1994; 33:685–706.

Chemotherapy

Chemotherapy 2001;47(suppl 3):9–14

Comparison of Side Effects of Levofloxacin versus Other Fluoroquinolones

Claude Carbon

Internal Medicine Unit, Bichat-Claude Bernard Hospital, Paris, France

Key Words

Fluoroquinolones · Levofloxacin · Safety · Adverse drug reactions · Toxicity · PMS data

Abstract

The side-effect profile of levofloxacin was compared with that of other fluoroquinolones based on European and international data from approximately 130 million prescriptions. Levofloxacin was found to be very safe with a low rate of hepatic abnormalities (1/650,000). In contrast, 140 trovafloxacin-treated patients developed hepatic problems, 14 of which were severe, and 8 required transplantation. The main CNS problems associated with fluoroquinolones include dizziness, convulsions, psychosis, and insomnia. Levofloxacin, ofloxacin, and moxifloxacin reportedly have the lowest potential of inducing central nervous system (CNS) adverse events among the fluoroquinolones currently available. Cardiovascular problems were seen in 1/15 million levofloxacin prescriptions compared to 1–3% of sparfloxacin patients having QTc prolongation of greater than 500 msec. Moxifloxacin was also associated with QTc prolongation when compared to non-fluoroquinolone comparators. Nausea, vomiting, and diarrhoea remain the main adverse drug reactions (ADRs) associated with levofloxacin. However, the ADR rate for levofloxacin is still one of the lowest of any fluoroquinolone at 2% (compared to 2–10% for other fluoroquinolones). Ofloxacin and levofloxacin have a very low phototoxic potential, whereas this is a problem for sparfloxacin, enoxacin, and pefloxacin. The tolerance profile of levofloxacin can be considered to be very good, and better than most, if not all of the fluoroquinolones available.

Introduction

Fluoroquinolones can now be characterised as one of the most important classes of antimicrobials available. Since their introduction, they have garnered a substantial share of

KARGER

Fax +41 61 306 12 34
E-Mail karger@karger.ch
www.karger.com

0009–3157/01/0479–0009$17.50/0

Accessible online at:
www.karger.com/journals/che

Claude Carbon, MD
Internal Medicine Unit, Bichat-Claude Bernard Hospital
46 Rue Henri Huchard
75877 Paris Cédex 18 (France)
Tel. +33 1 40 25 70 01, Fax +33 1 40 25 88 45

the infectious disease market. This has occurred over a number of years, as newer agents have become available. Due to alterations in their chemical structure, these new agents have gained extra bacterial potency across a wider spectrum of pathogens. While the earliest members of this class primarily had activity against Gram-negative bacteria, this has widened to encompass Gram-positive pathogens, as well as most of the important atypicals and anaerobes. In addition, the newer agents have an improved pharmacokinetic profile, resulting in better, more cost-effective administration schedules. Unfortunately, while most of the developments occurring among the fluoroquinolones have been positive, some agents have been associated with serious side effects. Such adverse events have led to a number of fluoroquinolones being removed from the market. This is particularly true for the compounds temafloxacin, trovafloxacin, grepafloxacin, clinafloxacin, and sparfloxacin. It is thus very important that a careful differentiation among the individual fluoroquinolones be carried out. This will allow the clinician to prescribe an agent which not only will be therapeutically effective, but one which will also be well tolerated and not associated with deleterious side effects. The following data helps to differentiate the new, safer fluoroquinolones from those that have higher adverse drug reaction (ADR) rates.

Earlier agents such as norfloxacin, ciprofloxacin, and ofloxacin have proven their safety with extended use over many years. In fact, ofloxacin has been used throughout the world in a very large number of patients, and during this time has been shown to be extremely safe. Ofloxacin contains two stereospecific isomers, a levo- and dextro-form. It is the levo-form that has been shown to possess the bacterial potency of ofloxacin, and based on this finding, levofloxacin was developed, which only contains the active isomer.

Table 1. Fluoroquinolone adverse events

Adverse event	Rate (%)
Gastrointestinal tract	0.8–6.8
CNS (serious)	0.9–4.7 (< 0.5)
Hypersensitivity	0.4–2.1
Phototoxicity	0.5–2.0
Cardiovascular	0.5–2.0
Renal/hepatic	0.5–4.5
Musculoskeletal	0.5–2.0

Adapted from reference 1.

Against this background, it is understandable that levofloxacin was heralded as a more effective fluoroquinolone, while possessing the safety profile of its parent compound. Levofloxacin received marketing approval in Japan in 1993, in the US in 1997, and more recently in Europe. It demonstrates essentially 100% bioavailability, and the 500-mg dose of levofloxacin is 5 times the unitary dose of ofloxacin, or 2.5 times the once-daily dose of ofloxacin. Thus, while there is a long history of ofloxacin use, it is necessary to assess what, if any, are the safety consequences of the higher concentrations of levofloxacin.

Evaluating the Safety Profiles

The side-effect profile of levofloxacin has been evaluated and compared with that of other fluoroquinolones, using European licensing approval data as well as results from a worldwide pharmacovigilance study. The European dossier included an evaluation of levofloxacin safety in more than 5,000 patients, while the international vigilance study incorporates results from approximately 130 million prescriptions. In 1999, Ball et al. [1] reported that adverse events associated with fluoroquinolones as a class range from 0.5%

Table 2. Adverse events from the European dossier

	Levofloxacin	Comparators
Number of patients	5,388 (40%)	3,528 (41%)
Drug-related adverse events	12%	13%
Early discontinuations	4%	5%
Severe adverse events	1%	1%

to almost 7%. Identification of specific problems reveals that gastrointestinal effects are the most common, occurring in 0.8–6.8%. The main ADRs of clinical concern are those of the central nervous system (CNS), which occur in 0.9–4.7% (although < 0.5% are deemed to be serious), cardiovascular effects (0.5–2.0%), renal and hepatic toxicity (0.5–4.5%), and phototoxicity (0.5–2.0%) (table 1).

Factors with the potential to influence the incidence of adverse events associated with levofloxacin were investigated in three double-blind trials, a comparison of 500 mg once daily versus 500 mg twice daily. This study showed no significant impact of dose on the rate of adverse events. Thus, doubling the dose of levofloxacin from 500 mg to 1,000 mg did not result in a corresponding increase in the incidence of side effects. When the 500 mg once-daily dose was further analysed it was shown that the incidence of ADRs was not dependent on age. In addition, there were no significant drug interactions noted, although the absorption of levofloxacin was impaired when administered with antacids or iron containing compounds.

European Dossier and Pharmacovigilance Data

European dossier data from 5,388 patients treated with levofloxacin was compared to data on other commonly used agents. These studies used a very wide, all-encompassing definition of side effects, resulting in a high rate for all agents tested. However, even in this situation, levofloxacin was shown to be as safe, or safer, than comparator agents. Results indicated that 12% of patients treated with levofloxacin developed an adverse event possibly related to the drug, but only 1% of these were classified as serious. Treatment with levofloxacin was discontinued in only 4%. In the comparator arm, 13% of more than 3,500 patients developed an adverse event, with 1% of these also classified as severe, and 5% of cases were discontinued due to adverse drug events (table 2). Thus, levofloxacin can be characterised as safe and unlikely to cause severe adverse events.

Table 3. Levofloxacin pharmacovigilance information

Tendinitis	1/500,000
Tendon rupture	1/1.6 million
Hepatic abnormalities	1/650,000
Anaphylactic reactions	1/1 million
Convulsions	1/1 million
Psychosis	1/6 million
Phototoxicity	1/12 million
Torsade de pointes	1/15 million

Supporting these results was very strong evidence from a huge pharmacovigilance study in which more than 130 million prescriptions for levofloxacin were registered (table 3). This study demonstrated that the probability for any serious side effects occurring with levofloxacin is minimal. Concern has been raised in the past about the effects of fluoroquinolones on joints and surrounding tissue. In particular, fluoroquinolones are not indicated for paediatric use, as the joint problems only seem to develop in young animals and children. Investigation of this side effect revealed that tendinitis occurred in 1/500,000 levofloxacin prescriptions, with tendon rupture only in 1/1.6 million prescriptions. Hence, this is clearly not a significant problem associated with levofloxacin.

The same study provided incidence rates for all of the major areas where fluoroquinolones seem likely to result in problems. For example, there is growing recognition that some fluoroquinolones cause hepatotoxicity. To show that this is not the case for levofloxacin, results from the same study revealed that hepatic abnormalities occurred in 1/650,000 levofloxacin prescriptions. There is also concern that fluoroquinolones may be associated with a class effect on the CNS, via γ-aminobutyric acid (GABA) binding. This can lead to convulsions and other CNS adverse events. Levofloxacin was shown to be safe in this regard with psychosis occurring in only 1/6 million prescriptions. Anaphylactic reactions are also rare, developing in only 1 patient for every million prescriptions. Phototoxicity has also been reported as a class effect associated with fluoroquinolones, but this only developed in 1/12 million prescriptions. Finally, cardiovascular problems, such as torsade de pointes, were very infrequent with levofloxacin, only seen in 1/15 million prescriptions. These data are very reliable, and important, as they are based upon such a large cohort of patients.

Not only do these data confirm the safety of levofloxacin, but they are also useful in comparing it to the other fluoroquinolones. For example, major ADRs have been demonstrated for other fluoroquinolones within a very short time frame, after far fewer prescriptions. More than 130 million prescriptions of levofloxacin were registered in the pharmacovigilance study. In contrast, temafloxacin was withdrawn for severe haemolytic–uremic syndrome after only 185,000 prescriptions. Trovafloxacin was withdrawn for serious hepatotoxicity, and grepafloxacin for serious cardiac events, after 2.5 and 2.65 million prescriptions, respectively. Therefore, the probability of serious side effects with levofloxacin appears to be negligible.

Gastrointestinal and Hepatic Adverse Events — How the Individual Fluoroquinolones Differ

Nausea, vomiting, and diarrhoea remain the main ADRs associated with levofloxacin. However, the ADR rate for levofloxacin is still one of the lowest of any fluoroquinolone at 2% (compared to 2–10% for other fluoroquinolones). These effects are usually benign, and severe diarrhoea with levofloxacin has only been reported at a rate of 1/3.6 million prescriptions.

The likelihood of hepatic toxicity occurring with individual fluoroquinolones appears to be related to the extent to which they undergo hepatic metabolism. In this regard, levofloxacin would not be expected to cause significant hepatic problems, as it has only minimal metabolism in the liver, but rather is excreted almost entirely through the renal system. In contrast, other fluoroquinolones undergo significant hepatic transformation, resulting in the production of a number of metabolites. The hepatic safety of levofloxacin is borne out by studies showing no liver abnormalities detectable among animals receiving levofloxacin. In addition, clinical results are supportive, demonstrating that less than 1%

of levofloxacin-treated patients develop any abnormal liver function tests. In contrast, other fluoroquinolones are associated with a 2–3% incidence rate of altered liver function tests. Highlighting the problems created by other fluoroquinolones causing hepatic adverse events are the recent problems associated with trovafloxacin that have led to its removal from the market. One hundred and forty patients treated with trovafloxacin for 28 days developed hepatic problems, with 9% having a greater than three-fold normal increase in their transaminase, with 14 severe cases of liver injury, of which 8 required transplantation. A retrospective review of animal data also detected a disturbance in some animals following administration of trovafloxacin. Against this, levofloxacin appears to be very safe.

Fluoroquinolones and Cardiovascular Adverse Events

The importance of cardiovascular abnormalities has also been increasingly recognised. The principal effect appears to be prolongation of the corrected QT (QTc) interval, and this may be a class effect, although the degree to which individual agents are affected may vary widely. There are two accepted definitions of QTc prolongation. First, an actual QTc value of more than 500 ms, or secondly, a greater than 60 ms increase compared to the normal value found in that patient. Using the first definition, it has been found that 1–3% of patients treated with sparfloxacin had QTc prolongation of more than 500 ms. In sharp contrast to this is data showing that such QTc prolongation only occurs in 1/15 million prescriptions for levofloxacin. Moxifloxacin has also been associated with QTc prolongation of more than 60 ms compared to non-fluoroquinolone comparators. The QTc prolongation can result in torsade de pointes, which has been reported for both sparfloxacin and grepafloxacin. At present, it is recommended that physicians monitor patients for this potential effect, especially if a high fluoroquinolone dose is given, or if the patient is already receiving other agents at the same time that are capable of prolonging QTc interval or are associated with other cardiac effects.

Defining the Agents Which Are More Likely to Result in Phototoxicity

In the past, phototoxicity has been one of the main adverse events associated with fluoroquinolones of concern to clinicians. Actual lesions can range from mild reddening through to serious photosensitivity and blister formation. Phototoxicity develops following the generation of free oxygen radicals under exposure to ultraviolet-A light. This can result in significant problems, and restriction in quality of life. As such, it is seen as a definite problem by patients, particularly among light-skinned patients and in areas with strong sun exposure. Therefore, a better understanding and clarification of the specific structure–adverse event profiles of the fluoroquinolones has focused on which substituents are likely to cause this problem. It has become apparent that phototoxicity is more likely to occur when 8-halogenated fluoroquinolones are prescribed. Investigation into this effect has led to the use of very well validated models to predict the risk of phototoxicity. These models have shown that ofloxacin and levofloxacin are well tolerated, with a very low phototoxic potential. However, there is a four-fold increased risk of phototoxicity developing following lomefloxacin administration, and this is even higher for sparfloxacin, enoxacin, and pefloxacin.

Convulsions — Not All Fluoroquinolones Are Responsible

Among the most worrying of the adverse events associated with fluoroquinolones are those that result in CNS changes. The main CNS problems reported by patients taking fluoroquinolones include dizziness, convulsions, psychosis and insomnia. The development of these effects seems to be related to the degree to which the fluoroquinolones bind to the GABA receptor, and their differing potential to act as GABA antagonists and bind to the *N*-methyl-D-aspartate receptor. Investigations into these effects have also shown them to be much more likely to occur when the patient is taking nonsteroidal anti-inflammatory agents (NSAIDs) at the same time. The effect of concomitant NSAID administration varies widely among individual fluoroquinolones. Some of the fluoroquinolones cause a dramatic increase in seizures when taken with NSAIDs, while others show a much-reduced change, with little effect from concomitant NSAID use. Levofloxacin administration is not associated with a high incidence of seizures, and this does not increase significantly when levofloxacin is prescribed at the same time as NSAIDs. Levofloxacin, ofloxacin, and moxifloxacin have been shown in rat hippocampal studies to have the lowest potential to induce CNS adverse events among the fluoroquinolones currently available.

Differences in Incidence of Other Adverse Events among the Fluoroquinolones

Tendinitis and tendon rupture represent a class effect, although there is a higher risk with pefloxacin. Risk factors for this occurring include age, corticosteroid use, renal disease, haemodialysis and transplantation. The incidence is low with ofloxacin, levofloxacin, ciprofloxacin and moxifloxacin. For levofloxacin, there have been 8 cases of tendinitis reported among 5,388 patients, with 4 related to the drug administration. Tendinitis with rupture was very rare, occurring in only 1/1.6 million prescriptions.

Renal toxicity is also very rare and represented mainly by crystalluria, for which there is a very significant role of alkaline urinary pH. Clinical trials of levofloxacin detected only three patients who developed acute renal failure following levofloxacin administration (0.06% versus 0.08% for comparators), with one case of acute renal failure for every 1.6 million prescriptions.

Conclusions

Levofloxacin is one of the most important of the new fluoroquinolones, with increased activity against Gram-positives including *Streptococcus pneumoniae*. This has resulted in levofloxacin firmly establishing a role for itself as a 'respiratory' fluoroquinolone. The tolerance profile of levofloxacin can be considered very good, and better than most, if not all, of the other fluoroquinolones available. Long-term experience with this agent indicates that it is unlikely that any unusual or unexpected events will occur, and the clinician can use the agent safely in most situations. It is recommended that care be exercised when using a higher dose (500 mg twice daily) in certain patients.

Reference

1 Ball P, Mandell L, Niki Y, Tillotson G: Comparative tolerability of the newer fluoroquinolone antibacterials. Drug Saf 1999;21:401–421.

Chemotherapy

Chemotherapy 2001;47(suppl 3):15–23

A Comparison of Side Effects of Levofloxacin to Other Agents Concerning the Ecological and Microbiological Effects on Normal Human Flora

Jacques F. Acar

Laboratoires de Microbiologie Médicale, Fondation Hôpital Saint-Joseph, Paris, France

Key Words
Fluoroquinolones · Cephalosporins · Macrolides · Amoxicillin–clavulanic acid · Levofloxacin · Resistance · Ecology

Abstract
The safety of levofloxacin was compared to that of non-fluoroquinolone alternatives used for respiratory tract infections. Results from five randomised controlled trials revealed that the incidence of any adverse events possibly associated with levofloxacin ranged from 5.8% to 22.7%, whereas that of comparators (ceftriaxone, cefuroxime axetil, clarithromycin and amoxicillin–clavulanic acid) ranged from 8.5% to 39.3%. The rate of adverse drug reactions (ADRs) was lower for levofloxacin in all trials. The most common adverse events for all agents tended to be gastrointestinal in nature. Levofloxacin was associated with a mild effect on the normal microflora, reaching a maximum at four days of therapy, with complete recovery being achieved by seven days post-therapy. No colonisation with resistant strains was observed during the period of levofloxacin therapy. Amoxicillin–clavulanic acid administration selected for resistant strains of Enterobacteriaceae, and ampicillin administration was associated with both resistant strains of Enterobacteriacae as well as *Candida* spp. Ceftriaxone selected resistant strains of *Clostridium difficile* and *Candida* spp. Thus, microflora effects favoured levofloxacin over all of the agents tested, including macrolides and tetracyclines. These results confirm that the ecological impact of levofloxacin is markedly less than that associated with non-fluoroquinolone comparators.

KARGER

Fax + 41 61 306 12 34
E-Mail karger@karger.ch
www.karger.com

0009–3157/01/0479–0015$17.50/0

Accessible online at:
www.karger.com/journals/che

Jacques F. Acar, MD
Laboratoire de Microbiologie Médicale
Fondation Hôpital Saint-Joseph
185, rue Raymond Losserand, 75674 Paris Cedex 14 (France)
Tel. +33 1 44 12 33 66, Fax +33 1 44 12 34 93

Introduction

Fluoroquinolones are now widely recognised to be an excellent treatment option for managing a wide range of infections. While earlier agents in this class, such as norfloxacin, ciprofloxacin, and ofloxacin, were primarily effective against aerobic organisms, particularly Gram-negative bacteria, the newer agents, exemplified by levofloxacin, moxifloxacin, and gatifloxacin, have a broader spectrum of antimicrobial activity. In addition to covering the previous pathogens, these newer agents also possess activity against Gram-positive bacteria and many clinically relevant anaerobes.

With the fluoroquinolones increasing in use, and the majority of newer agents in this class possessing this increased spectrum of antibacterial potency, it has become important to look at factors which the clinician can use to help decide which antibiotic to use when treating specific patients. When selecting an antimicrobial agent, it is important to consider not only the proven efficacy, but also to look at other factors such as adverse event profiles and cost. Adverse events themselves can be classified as direct effects, as exerted on body systems, or indirect effects, such as those arising from the ecological impact an agent has on normal intestinal flora. These factors can be used to differentiate between different classes of antimicrobials, as well as between individual agents within a class. This is becoming even more important, as it is apparent that there are marked differences among the fluoroquinolones concerning their probability of causing adverse events. It is also necessary to differentiate between fluoroquinolones and other classes of agents in terms of adverse events. This is the focus of this paper.

Randomised Controlled Trials Comparing Levofloxacin with Other Agents

In the past, assessment of adverse effects associated with fluoroquinolones has not been an integral part of many studies, and there is little data available that can reliably differentiate among these compounds. For a comparison between levofloxacin and non-fluoroquinolone alternatives used in the treatment of respiratory tract infections (RTIs) to be accurate and reliable, data from blinded controlled studies are needed, with the number of patients treated with levofloxacin and other agents comparable. Five studies fulfil these criteria, and results from these are used to contrast the safety profile of levofloxacin against that of other commonly used agents in the treatment of RTIs [1–5].

The studies were performed from 1997 to 1999. The first study, performed by File et al. [1], compared intravenous and/or oral levofloxacin 500 mg versus ceftriaxone and/or cefuroxime axetil in patients with community-acquired pneumonia (CAP). Five hundred and eighty-four out of 590 patients enrolled in the study were to be evaluated for safety. Most of the adverse events reported were mild. Seventeen patients treated with levofloxacin (5.8%) were assessed as having a possible or definite drug related event. In comparison, 8.5% of the ceftriaxone/cefuroxime axetil group developed adverse events.

In this study, 25 patients stopped taking the drug due to side effects (13 with levofloxacin, 12 with ceftriaxone/cefuroxime axetil giving a discontinuation rate of 5.7% for levofloxacin and 5.2% for the comparator). Most of the discontinuations in both groups were due to gastrointestinal (GI) complaints.

In a 1998 study by Norrby et al. [2], 500 mg levofloxacin twice daily was compared to ceftriaxone. In this study, 22% of

Table 1. Incidence of gastrointestinal side effects in randomised controlled trials

Study	Symptoms	Levofloxacin	Ceftriaxone and/or cefuroxime axetil	Ceftriaxone
File et al. [1]	GI complaints	1.7%	4.0%	–
	Diarrhoea	1.4%	3.8%	–
Norrby et al. [2]	GI complaints	4.8%	–	6.9%
	Diarrhoea	1.9%	–	4.6%

levofloxacin-treated patients developed some form of possibly related adverse drug reaction (ADR). In comparison, 26% of the ceftriaxone group were reported to have ADRs. Another 1998 study by Lasko et al. [3] compared levofloxacin with clarithromycin. In this study, the rate of ADRs for levofloxacin was 22% compared to a higher 30% for the clarithromycin group. Finally, the first of two studies performed by Adelglass et al. [4] compared levofloxacin with clarithromycin, and reported a 14.8% incidence rate of ADRs for levofloxacin compared to 24.8% for the comparator. In the second study [5], 21.2% of patients treated with amoxicillin–clavulanic acid (125 mg t.i.d.) developed possible ADRs compared to 7.4% in the levofloxacin group.

Thus, among these five trials, the incidence of any adverse event that could possibly be associated with levofloxacin ranged from 5.8% to 22%. The incidence of ADRs was lower for levofloxacin compared to the other agents in all trials represented, with their total ADR rate ranging from 8.5% to 39%. Throughout the trials, the discontinuation rate related to ADRs in the levofloxacin groups was 1.8–5.7%, a rate similar to those of the comparators (1.8–7%). The rate of serious side effects was similar for both groups. The enormous differences reported by the individual studies reflect the different doses used and the classification of ADRs.

Gastrointestinal Adverse Events Are the Most Common

The most common adverse events for all agents tended to be GI in nature, with these symptoms occurring in 1.7% of patients treated with levofloxacin compared to 4.0% for ceftriaxone and/or cefuroxime axetil. Nausea was the most common problem, occurring in 1.7%, followed by diarrhoea (1.4%), and injection site pain (1.0%). The most common adverse events related to the comparator group were GI complaints in 4.0%, followed by diarrhoea (3.8%), nausea (2.0%), dyspepsia (1.0%), and vomiting (1.0%) [1]. Diarrhoea is clearly less frequent with levofloxacin than ceftriaxone/cefuroxime axetil, which is to be expected given that ceftriaxone is mainly eliminated through the bowel, creating a change in the intestinal flora. Confirmation of these results came from the study by Norrby et al. [2], which also compared levofloxacin to ceftriaxone. Again, the rate of GI complaints was less for levofloxacin than the comparator (4.8% versus 6.9%), and diarrhoea was much more common with ceftriaxone at 4.6% compared to only 1.9% with levofloxacin (table 1).

The superiority of levofloxacin in terms of a lower rate of GI side effects was confirmed in the study by Adelglass et al. [5], which compared levofloxacin with amoxicillin–clavu-

Table 2. Incidence of gastrointestinal side effects in randomised controlled trials

Study	Symptoms	Levofloxacin	Amoxicillin–clavulanic acid
Adelglass et al. [2]	Nausea	1.7%	4.0%
	Abdominal pain	1.0%	1.7%
	Flatulence	0.3%	1.3%
	Vomiting	0%	1.7%
	Diarrhoea	1.3%	11.6%

Table 3. Incidence of gastrointestinal side effects in randomised controlled trials

Study	Symptoms	Levofloxacin	Clarithromycin
Adelglass et al. [4]	Nausea	5.6%	6.5%
	Abdominal pain	1.9%	3.7%
	Diarrhoea	0.9%	5.6%
	Taste perversion	0.9%	12.0%
Lasko et al. [3]	GI disorder	16.7%	33.3%
	Taste perversion	0.8%	7.7%

lanic acid. In this trial, the comparator agent was associated with 4.0% of patients experiencing nausea, 1.7% complaining of abdominal pain, 1.3% flatulence, and 1.7% vomiting. In contrast, levofloxacin results were 1.7% nausea, 1.0% abdominal pain, 0.3% flatulence, and no cases of vomiting. Diarrhoea was also much more marked in the amoxicillin–clavulanic acid group, with 11.6% of these patients developing this problem, compared to a much lower 1.3% in the levofloxacin group (table 2).

The second study by Adelglass et al. [4], which compared twice-daily 500 mg clarithromycin with levofloxacin 500 mg once daily, found that levofloxacin was much more well tolerated. Results from this trial confirmed that nausea occurred in 5.6% of levofloxacin patients compared to 6.5% in the comparator. Only 0.9% of patients experienced diarrhoea with levofloxacin, compared to 5.6% in the clarithromycin arm. This was confirmed in the study by Lasko et al. [3] comparing levofloxacin and clarithromycin, where the overall incidence of GI disorders with levofloxacin was reported to be 16.7% compared to 33.3% in the clarithromycin group (table 3). Both studies revealed that taste perversion was a noted adverse event associated with clarithromycin (7.7–12%), but was negligible in the levofloxacin arm (0.8–0.9%). In general, candidiasis developed with a frequency of 1.0–2.0%, which was comparable among the antibiotics, except amoxicillin–clavulanic acid, which was associated with a much higher incidence of candidiasis after therapy (7%).

Four of the five studies also evaluated the incidence of central nervous system (CNS) adverse events. In the study by Norrby et al. [2], 2.2% of levofloxacin treated patients developed dizziness, insomnia, or headache. In contrast, 1.3% of the ceftriaxone treated patients reported this problem. In the study by Lasko et al. [3], 6.7% of levofloxacin patients developed CNS problems possibly related to levofloxacin, compared to 4.3% in the clarithromycin group. The other study versus clarithromycin reported a rate of 2.8% for CNS effects in those treated with clarithromycin compared to 3.7% in the levofloxacin arm [4]. Finally, 0.3% of amoxicillin–clavulanic acid treated patients developed headache, dizziness, or insomnia compared to 0.6% in the levofloxacin arm. There were no statistically significant differences between levofloxacin and any of the other comparators in terms of causing CNS effects.

Ecological Effects of Antimicrobial Administration — Does This Lead to Resistance?

There is growing interest in the effect of antibiotics on the normal microflora, as it becomes apparent that colonisation by resistant mutants is more likely following GI ecological changes associated with antibiotic treatment. Such treatment can have numerous effects on the normal microflora — this can be related to changes in the species present, the days of treatment needed for these ecological effects to develop, and the number of days needed to recover after discontinuation of treatment. In addition, selection of resistant strains among the baseline species and colonisation with new resistant species are now seen as possible outcomes following antibiotic treatment, and the extent of this may relate to the age of the patient and the location in the GI system where the ecological impact is most apparent.

To investigate the ecological effects on the normal oral and intestinal flora following levofloxacin administration, a study was undertaken among normal volunteers [6]. Subjects received a seven-day course of 500 mg levofloxacin. In the intestinal flora, *Enterococcus* spp. and *Escherichia coli* were noted to decrease after the fourth day of treatment, and following cessation of treatment, it took almost 7 days to return to normal levels (fig. 1). During the same period, there was no change in yeast and bacillus levels associated with levofloxacin treatment (fig. 1). When looking at anaerobes, an unexpected decrease in *Clostridium* spp. was noted on the fourth day, reaching its maximum decrease on day 7 and then returning to normal by day 14. Levels of *Bacteroides* spp., *Bifidobacterium* spp. and *Lactobacillus* spp. were relatively unchanged (fig. 2). In the normal oral flora, the total amount of *Streptococcus* spp. remained stable, although there was a decrease in the percentage of *Streptococcus mitior* present. During levofloxacin therapy, *Neisseria* spp. were eliminated and *Peptostreptococcus* spp. were partly suppressed. No colonisation with resistant strains was observed during the period of levofloxacin therapy.

Clarifying the Effects on Normal Gastrointestinal Flora — Levofloxacin versus Other Agents

The effect on normal GI microflora caused by other agents (ampicillin, amoxicillin–clavulanic acid, ceftriaxone, cefuroxime axetil, cefixime, imipenem, clarithromycin, clindamycin, doxycycline, norfloxacin, and ofloxacin) was investigated and extensively reviewed by Edlund and Nord [7] (tables 4, 5).

When comparing results, most agents had a similar effect on aerobic Gram-positive cocci and anaerobes. One study by Motohiro et al. [8] showed an increase of Enterobacteriaceae with amoxicillin–clavulanic acid in 4 subjects. Ampicillin administration was asso-

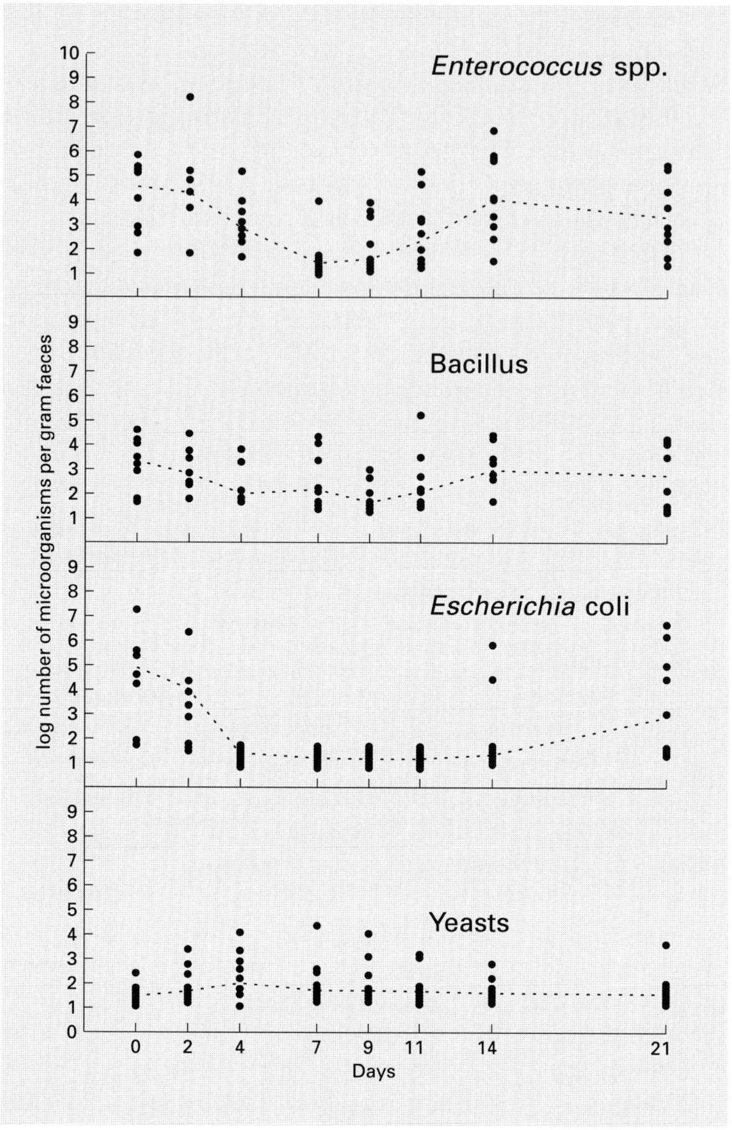

Fig. 1. Impact of levofloxacin on the aerobic intestinal microflora of 10 volunteers receiving 500 mg levofloxacin perorally once daily for 7 days (––– = median log value). Adapted from reference 6.

ciated with both resistant strains of *Enterobacteriacae* spp. as well as *Candida* spp. It was also found that while ceftriaxone had an effect comparable to levofloxacin on the intestinal microflora, it was adversely associated with the selection of resistant strains of *Clostridium difficile* and *Candida* spp.

Clindamycin treatment resulted in resistant stains of *C. difficile*, and doxycycline was associated with colonisation by resistant *Candida* spp. Thus, microflora effects favoured levofloxacin. Ofloxacin and levofloxacin treatment caused no colonisation of the normal microflora with resistant strains. This is a

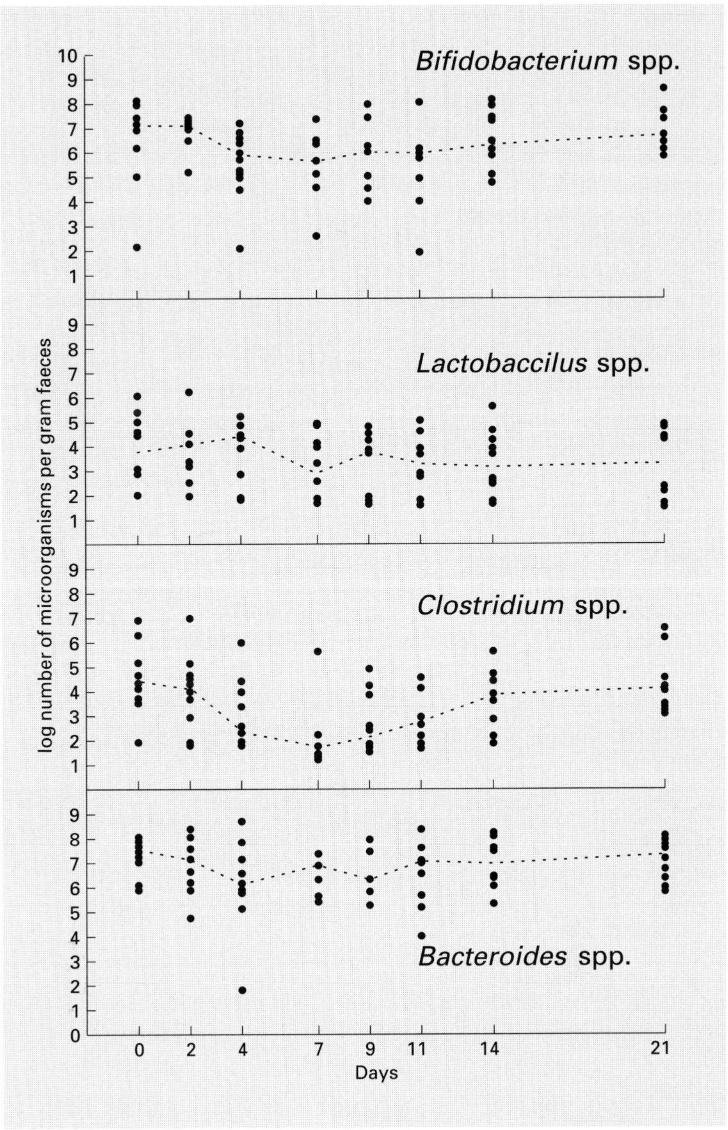

Fig. 2. Impact of levofloxacin on the anaerobic intestinal microflora of 10 volunteers receiving 500 mg levofloxacin perorally once daily for 7 days (--- = median log value). Adapted from reference 6.

clinical benefit of levofloxacin, demonstrating a potential to be associated with less resistance. This advantageous feature possessed by levofloxacin, along with its more favourable tolerability profile compared to other nonfluoroquinolone respiratory agents, make it a useful drug that the clinician can rely on.

Conclusion

Patients exhibited excellent tolerance to levofloxacin (500 mg once or twice daily), which was generally associated with fewer side effects than the comparator agents, ceftriaxone, cefuroxime axetil, clarithromycin,

Table 4. Effect of antibiotics on gastrointestinal flora

Antibiotics	Enterobacter spp.	Aerobic Gram-positive cocci	Anaerobes	Resistant strains		
				Enterobacter spp.	*Clostridium difficile*	*Candida* spp.
Ampicillin	↓	↓	↓	+	–	+
Amoxicillin–clavulanic acid	↑	↓	↓	+	–	–
Ceftriaxone	↓↓	↓	↓	–	+	+
Cefuroxime axetil	↓	↓	↓	–	–	+
Cefixime	↓	↑	↓↓	–	+	–
Imipenem	↓	–	↓↓	–	–	–
Levofloxacin	↓↓	↓	↓	–	–	–

Adapted from reference 7.

Table 5. Effect of antibiotics on gastrointestinal flora [3]

Antibiotics	*Enterobacter* spp.	Aerobic Gram-positive cocci	Anaerobes	Resistant strains		
				Enterobacter spp.	*Clostridium difficile*	*Candida* spp.
Clarithromycin	↓	↓	–	–	–	–
Clindamycin	–	↑	↓↓	–	+	–
Doxycycline	↓	↓	–	+	–	+
Norfloxacin	↓↓	–	–	–	–	–
Ofloxacin	↓↓	↓	↓	–	–	–
Levofloxacin	↓↓	↓	↓	–	–	–

Adapted from reference 7.

and amoxicillin–clavulanic acid. Adverse events occurred relatively rarely and further surveillance is required to confirm the low ADR rates. Levofloxacin was associated with a mild effect on the normal GI microflora, reaching a maximum at 4 days of therapy and complete recovery was achieved by 7 days post-therapy. In contrast to comparator agents, there was no evidence of colonisation with resistant strains following levofloxacin treatment. These results confirm that the ecological impact of levofloxacin is markedly less than that associated with non-fluoroquinolone comparators, making this agent one of the most preferred of those currently available for treating RTIs.

References

1 File TM Jr, Segreti J, Dunbar L, Player R, Kohler R, Williams RR, Kojak C, Rubin A: A multicenter, randomized study comparing the efficacy and safety of intravenous and/or oral levofloxacin versus ceftriaxone and/or cefuroxime axetil in treatment of adults with community-acquired pneumonia. Antimicrob Agents Chemother 1997;41:1965–1972.

2 Norrby SR, Petermann W, Willcox PA, Vetter N, Salewski E: A comparative study of levofloxacin and ceftriaxone in the treatment of hospitalized patients with pneumonia. Scand J Infect Dis 1998;30:397–404.

3 Lasko B, Lau CY, Saint-Pierre C, Reddington JL, Martel A, Anstey RJ: Efficacy and safety of oral levofloxacin compared with clarithromycin in the treatment of acute sinusitis in adults: A multicentre, double-blind, randomized study. The Canadian Sinusitis Study Group. J Int Med Res 1998;26:281–291.

4 Adelglass J, Jones TM, Ruoff G, Kahn JB, Wiesinger BA, Rielly-Gauvin K, Siu CO: A multicenter, investigator-blinded, randomized comparison of oral levofloxacin and oral clarithromycin in the treatment of acute bacterial sinusitis. Pharmacotherapy 1998;18:1255–1263.

5 Adelglass J, DeAbate CA, McElvaine P, Fowler CL, LoCocco J, Campbell T: Comparison of the effectiveness of levofloxacin and amoxicillin–clavulanate for the treatment of acute sinusitis in adults. Otolaryngol Head Neck Surg 1999;120:320–327.

6 Edlund C, Sjöstedt S, Nord CE: Comparative effects of levofloxacin and ofloxacin on the normal oral and intestinal microflora. Scand J Infect Dis 1997;29:383–386.

7 Edlund C, Nord CE: Ecological impact of antimicrobial agents on human intestinal microflora. Alpe Adria Microbiol J 1993;3:137–164.

8 Motohiro T, Tanaka K, Koga T, Shimada Y, Tomita N, Sakata Y, Fujimoto T, Nishiyama T, Kuda N, Ishimoto K, Tominaga K, Tamashita F: Effect of BRL 25000 (clavulanic acid–amoxicillin) on bacterial flora in human feces. Jpn J Antibiot 1985;38:441–480.

Chemotherapy

Chemotherapy 2001;47(suppl 3):24–31

Evidence of Different Profiles of Side Effects and Drug–Drug Interactions among the Quinolones — The Pharmacokinetic Standpoint

Hartmut Lode

Department of Chest and Infectious Diseases, Emil von Behring Hospital, Department Heckeshorn, Berlin, Germany

Key Words

Fluoroquinolones · Levofloxacin · Safety · ADRs · Pharmacokinetics · Drug–drug interactions

Abstract

Recent pharmacokinetic data, interaction profiles, and specific tolerance problems associated with the fluoroquinolones are reviewed. Oral absorption was highest for levofloxacin (99–100%), and 500 mg oral levofloxacin achieved a much higher initial concentration than either sparfloxacin (400 mg) or ciprofloxacin (500 mg, b.i.d.), with a slow drop in concentration over 24 h. The C_{max} achieved after an oral 250-mg dose ranged from a low of 1.2 μg/ml/70 kg for ciprofloxacin, to 1.71 for gatifloxacin and 2.17 for moxifloxacin, to a high of 2.48 for levofloxacin ($p <$ 0.01). Ciprofloxacin had the lowest AUC of 4.6 μg/ml/70 kg, gatifloxacin 15, levofloxacin 17.9, and moxifloxacin 19.7 μg/ml/70 kg ($p <$ 0.01). All fluoroquinolones interact with multivalent cation-containing products and bioavailability is reduced by 50% when coadministered with iron compounds (ciprofloxacin and moxifloxacin are more affected than levofloxacin or gemifloxacin). The interaction between theophylline and fluoroquinolones is most marked with enoxacin, pefloxacin, and ciprofloxacin, with no such interaction reported for levofloxacin. Sparfloxacin is associated with cardiac manifestations of QTc prolongation and has a high phototoxicity potential. Moxifloxacin is currently under observation concerning QTc effects. Levofloxacin has no QTc prolongation and a very low phototoxic potential, making it one of the safest new fluoroquinolones.

KARGER

Fax + 41 61 306 12 34
E-Mail karger@karger.ch
www.karger.com

0009–3157/01/0479–0024$17.50/0

Accessible online at:
www.karger.com/journals/che

Hartmut Lode, MD, City Hospital Berlin-H-Heckeshorn
Laboratory for Chemotherapy and Immunology, Department of Chest and Infectious Diseases, Zum Heckeshorn 33, Main Building
D–14109 Berlin (Germany), Tel. +49 30 80 02 22 23
Fax +49 30 80 02 26 23, E-Mail haloheck@zedat.fu-berlin.de

Introduction

The newer fluoroquinolones, often called 'respiratory' fluoroquinolones, have been substantially improved since the introduction of their earlier forerunners. The latest agents available have an expanded spectrum of activity covering a wide range of pathogens, including many organisms resistant to other antimicrobials. In order to differentiate among these new improved fluoroquinolones, it is important to look at basic pharmacological principles. In this regard, pharmacokinetic features have been increasingly used to discriminate among individual quinolones, allowing the clinician to select the best agent, and to administer it in the most optimal schedule. The following article reports on three major aspects of fluoroquinolone pharmacology. First, it outlines the recent data highlighting the different pharmacokinetic features possessed by each fluoroquinolone. Second, the interaction profiles are described both for older agents such as ciprofloxacin and ofloxacin, as well as for newer agents. Third, it addresses specific tolerance problems associated with some of the latest fluoroquinolones.

Pharmacokinetic Differences among the Fluoroquinolones Clarified

Since their introduction, there has been increasing data available on the pharmacokinetic properties of the various fluoroquinolones. Studies investigating these features have included results in healthy volunteers, patients with various bacterial infections, as well as patients with specific factors such as old age and reduced renal or hepatic function. A number of reviews have highlighted the pharmacokinetic features of individual agents.

Absorption

All of the fluoroquinolones have good oral absorption from the gastrointestinal tract. However, even at this basic level there are differences among individual agents. It is well recognised that levofloxacin, one of the newer fluoroquinolones, has the best gastrointestinal absorption, achieving 99–100% bioavailability when administered orally. Differences in absorption relate to the lipophilic properties of the fluoroquinolones. Low lipophilic agents have an absorption rate of about 50–70%, while agents such as levofloxacin with medium lipophilic properties exert extremely good bioavailability rates of essentially 100%. The bioavailability of both ciprofloxacin and grepafloxacin is approximately 70%, whereas it is 87% for trovafloxacin, and 92% for sparfloxacin [1]. The only other agent that comes near to the high levels of gastrointestinal absorption of levofloxacin is gatifloxacin with a 98% oral bioavailability rate. Although absorption of levofloxacin may be slightly delayed when taken with food, the overall bioavailability is not affected. This makes it possible to administer the same dose of levofloxacin either orally or intravenously, which is not a feature possessed by any other fluoroquinolone.

Assessment of half-life ($t_{1/2}$) has also revealed differences between the various fluoroquinolones. In a study of 12 volunteers, levofloxacin, ciprofloxacin, trovafloxacin, moxifloxacin and gatifloxacin were administered at their usual doses. Levofloxacin achieved the highest serum concentration, with the value slowly reducing over the subsequent 48 h ($t_{1/2}$ 6.8–7.6 h) [2]. The other new fluoroquinolones had a similar pharmacokinetic profile, but the concentration of ciprofloxacin dissipated much more quickly (fig. 1). Levofloxacin possesses the advantageous feature of a long elimination time, while ciprofloxacin

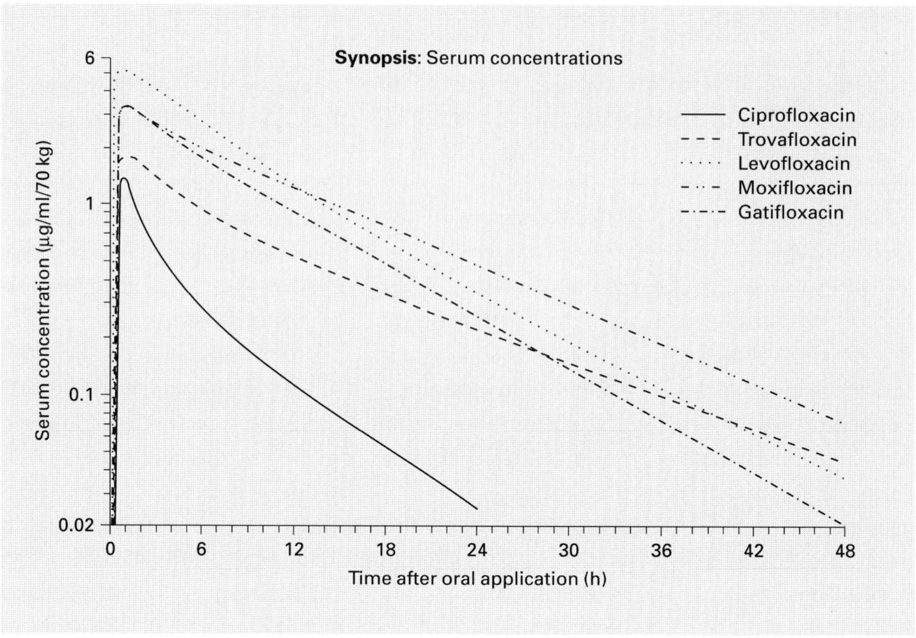

Fig. 1. Mean serum concentrations of selected fluoroquinolones. Adapted from reference 2.

has a relatively short elimination, necessitating twice-daily administration schedules. These differences result in levofloxacin being a very active agent when administered in a cost-effective once-daily schedule. These results were confirmed in a study by Chien et al. [3], which demonstrated that levofloxacin given at an oral dose of 500 mg achieved a much higher initial concentration than either sparfloxacin (400 mg) or ciprofloxacin (500 mg b.i.d.), and that it had a slow sustained drop in concentration over 24 h.

C_{max}, AUC, and Other Pharmacological Parameters

Previous studies have demonstrated that fluoroquinolones, as an antimicrobial class, exert their killing effect in a concentration-dependent manner. Therefore, the peak concentration (C_{max}) that they attain is the most important factor associated with their efficacy, rather than time above the minimum inhibitory concentration (Time > MIC). Concentration-dependent killing, as performed by the fluoroquinolones, means that the kill rate at peak concentrations is greater than at concentrations near the middle of the curve, and that these middle values are also more likely to result in cell kill than lower concentrations close to the MIC. Thus, it is important when identifying features associated with individual fluoroquinolones to look at some of their basic pharmacokinetic data, primarily the maximum concentration they achieve. The C_{max} achieved after a single oral dose of 250 mg ranged from a low of 1.2 μg/ml/70 kg for ciprofloxacin to 1.71 μg/ml/70 kg for gatifloxacin, and 2.17 μg/ml/70 kg for moxifloxa-

Table 1. Pharmacokinetic data of selected fluoroquinolones

HPLC	C_{max} (μg/ml/70 kg)	AUC_{tot} (μg/ml/70 kg)
Ciprofloxacin	1.2 ± 0.341	4.6 ± 1.0
Gatifloxacin	1.71 ± 0.37*	15 ± 1.9*
Levofloxacin	2.48 ± 0.534*	17.9 ± 1.76*
Moxifloxacin	2.17 ± 0.805*	19.7 ± 2.67*
Trovafloxacin	2.09 ± 0.58*	19.5 ± 3.1*

Pharmacokinetic data normalised to an average dosage of 200 mg per fluoroquinolone per volunteer (mean ± SD).
* Differences between ciprofloxacin and the other four fluoroquinolones were significant ($p < 0.01$).
Adapted from reference 2.

cin, to a high of 2.48 μg/ml/70 kg for levofloxacin — a statistically significant benefit for levofloxacin ($p < 0.01$) (table 1) [2].

With regard to the area under the concentration–time curve (AUC), an important factor reflecting a drug's bioavailability, ciprofloxacin again had the lowest value of 4.6 μg/ml/70 kg. Data for this study was taken from volunteers, normalised to an average dose of 200 mg per fluoroquinolone. The AUC was 15 μg/ml/70 kg for gatifloxacin, 17.9 μg/ml/70 kg for levofloxacin, and 19.7 μg/ml/70 kg for moxifloxacin. Thus, the bioavailability of these latter three drugs is much higher than that for ciprofloxacin ($p < 0.01$) (table 1) [2].

Metabolism and Excretion

Following absorption, fluoroquinolones can be metabolised and excreted either through glucuronisation in the liver or oxidation utilising the P450 enzyme systems, followed by kidney elimination. If hepatic metabolism is the major route of metabolism, then there is a greater likelihood of metabolites being formed, resulting in more drug–drug interactions. It also means that for patients with reduced liver function, dosage adjustment is necessary. Administration of fluoroquinolones that undergo liver metabolisation is also more likely to result in disturbances in the intestinal bacterial flora. Such disturbances are now being seen to be associated with significant problems, which are described in the previous article in this supplement written by Prof. Acar. Drugs that undergo hepatic metabolisation include sparfloxacin, grepafloxacin, trovafloxacin, and moxifloxacin. Monitoring the concentration of these drugs should therefore be performed in patients with liver dysfunction. In contrast, norfloxacin, ofloxacin, ciprofloxacin, and levofloxacin are all eliminated through the kidney with very limited hepatic metabolism. Levofloxacin and gatifloxacin have a relatively high urinary elimination rate of over 70%, which drops to 40% for ciprofloxacin and 20% for moxifloxacin (fig. 2) [2]. This means that levofloxacin dosage should be monitored when used in patients with reduced renal activity.

Potential Fluoroquinolone–Drug Interactions

When first developed, the fluoroquinolones were systematically assessed for possible interactions among a number of agents. All of the agents were shown to interact with multivalent cation-containing products. Thus, all aluminium- or magnesium-containing antacids or calcium, iron, or zinc agents when used in combination with fluoroquinolones had a tremendous impact on bioavailability [4]. This is illustrated by a study in which fasting volunteers reached a maximum concentration of 1.8 μg/ml following 500 mg ciprofloxacin

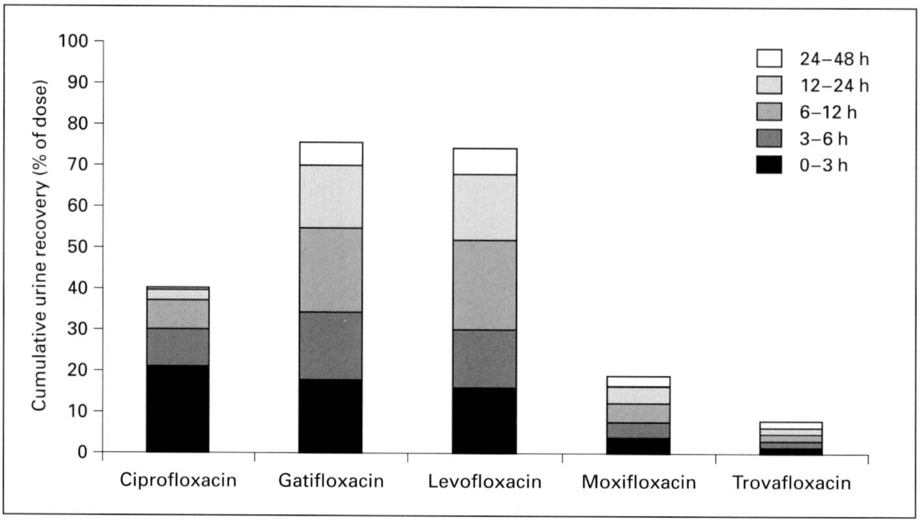

Fig. 2. Urinary elimination of selected fluoroquinolones. Adapted from reference 2.

administration. However, when this was given with antacids (Maalox®), the maximum concentration was dramatically reduced to 0.13 μg/ml [5]. While all fluoroquinolones are associated with this effect, there are differences among individual agents. For example, when the same study was done with 200 mg ofloxacin, the C_{max} was 2.2 μg/ml. When co-administered with antacids, the C_{max} reduced to 0.5 μg/ml, a much less pronounced decrease than that shown by ciprofloxacin. The interaction between fluoroquinolones and antacids is caused by chelation taking place when used together, leading to reduced oral bioavailability. This can be avoided if the antacid or similar compound is taken 4 h after the quinolone. While all agents have considerable interaction with aluminium-containing antacids, there are differences in the degree of interaction with calcium-containing antacids. The most pronounced effect in this situation is with ciprofloxacin, with a more limited effect occurring with other fluoroquinolones (table 2) [6]. Other gastrointestinal compounds implicated in fluoroquinolone interactions include ranitidine and sucralfate. Again, these relate to specific agents. For example, when ciprofloxacin was administered with ranitidine, the C_{max} dropped from 1.8 μg/ml to 1.7 μg/ml, but there was no drop in the C_{max} of ofloxacin when taken with ranitidine.

Fluoroquinolones also interact with sucralfate, via production of a chelate complex in the stomach, and again this is more marked with ciprofloxacin. Their bioavailability is also generally reduced by about 50% when co-administered with iron compounds, although ciprofloxacin and moxifloxacin are more affected by this interaction than either levofloxacin or gemifloxacin. Dairy products have been shown to reduce the absorption of ciprofloxacin to a greater extent than the newer agents.

The effect of food on gastrointestinal absorption has also been investigated in a study comparing the maximal serum concentration of ciprofloxacin and ofloxacin achieved when given alone or with food. Ten fasting volun-

Table 2. Drug and food interactions with selected fluoroquinolones

	Ciprofloxacin	Levofloxacin	Moxifloxacin	Gatifloxacin	Gemifloxacin
Absorption of the quinolones is affected when administered concomitantly with the following:					
Aluminium- or magnesium-containing antacids	↓↓↓	↓↓↓	↓↓↓	↓↓↓	↓↓↓
Calcium-containing antacids	↓↓	↓	↓	↓	?
Ferrous sulfate	↓↓↓	↓↓	↓↓↓	↓↓↓	↓↓
Sucralfate	↓↓↓↓	↓↓↓	↓↓↓	?	↓↓↓
Dairy products	↓↓	↓	↓	?	?
Food	↓	–	↓	?	↓

Modified from reference 6.

Table 3. Drug interactions with selected fluoroquinolones

	Ciprofloxacin	Levofloxacin	Moxifloxacin	Gatifloxacin	Gemifloxacin
Quinolones may interfere with the metabolism of the following:					
Increased level of					
Theophylline	↑↑	–	–	–	–
Caffeine	↑↑	–	?	?	?
Warfarin	slight to ↑	–	–	–	–

Modified from reference 6.

teers received 250 mg ciprofloxacin orally. When this was combined with a standard breakfast, the absorption was markedly reduced, with a serum concentration almost 50% lower than when given without food. In this study, the C_{max} reduced from 1.6 μg/ml to 0.9 μg/ml. In comparison, when 200 mg ofloxacin was given with food, the C_{max} dropped from 2.2 μg/ml to 1.7 μg/ml [7]. Other reports have also confirmed that the absorption of levofloxacin is not affected by food.

Drug–drug interactions can be a significant problem for some compounds. An investigation of this has shown that a clinically very important interaction occurs between fluoroquinolones and theophylline and other methylxanthines, such as caffeine. This interaction is most noticeable with enoxacin, pefloxacin, and ciprofloxacin, and is related to involvement in the cytochrome P450 system. This is of great concern when treating patients with respiratory tract infections, as a significant number of such people may also be on theophylline. While ciprofloxacin has a marked interaction with theophylline, reports of a similar but lesser problem with grepafloxacin have been presented. No such interaction has been reported for levofloxacin (table 3), nor does levofloxacin interact with caffeine. The potential for this interaction with moxifloxacin, gatifloxacin and gemifloxacin has not been fully investigated. It is impressive that there is

Table 4. Inhibition of I_{kr} currents in HERG channels

Concentration	Inhibition, % (mean ± SEM)			
	Ciprofloxacin	Gatifloxacin	Moxifloxacin	Sparfloxacin
10 μ*M*	5.1 ± 3.1	3.3 ± 1.5	10.3 ± 2.8	16.9 ± 3.7
30 μ*M*	6.3 ± 2.3	8.6 ± 3.4	20.5 ± 1.6	35.3 ± 3.6
100 μ*M*	11.1 ± 4.8	20.4 ± 6.0	37.8 ± 4.8	60.8 ± 3.4
300 μ*M*	16.6 ± 6.1	36.6 ± 7.7	59.2 ± 8.3	79.5 ± 3.6

Modified from reference 8.

no clinically significant interaction between levofloxacin and food, or between levofloxacin and any of the following frequently prescribed drugs: cyclosporine, digoxin, glibenclamide, probenecid, theophylline, and warfarin.

Safety of the Fluoroquinolones

Understanding the relationships between specific fluoroquinolone structures and the development of adverse events has rapidly increased over the last few years [4]. It is now known that the interaction with theophylline and genetic toxicity is associated with specific constituents at the R1 position, while R7 is involved in γ-aminobutyric acid (GABA) binding, interaction with non-steroidal anti-inflammatory drugs (NSAIDs), as well as theophylline interaction and genetic toxicity. Other important fluoroquinolone-induced toxicities include phototoxicity, cardiotoxicity, hepatotoxicity, neurotoxicity and effects on connective tissue.

Phototoxicity is a commonly described side effect associated with fluoroquinolones. This appears to be related to substitution at positions X8 and R5. Constituents at R5 listed in decreasing order for causing phototoxicity are $CH_3 \gg H > NH_2$. Among the individual agents, sparfloxacin has been identified as one of the most likely to cause phototoxicity. A small dose of 18 mg/kg has been demonstrated to cause photosensitivity. In contrast, ofloxacin and ciprofloxacin can both be given at a dose of greater than 300 mg/kg without causing phototoxicity. Ofloxacin has a very low phototoxic potential, and thus by association, this is also likely to be the case for levofloxacin.

A recent insight into the pathogenesis of cardiovascular side effects caused by fluoroquinolones is the role of alterations in myocardial transfer channels [8]. For example, the HERG channel, a potassium-transferring channel, is affected to differing degrees by individual fluoroquinolones. At low doses of the drugs, the percentage inhibition is highest for sparfloxacin, but as the dosage of the agent increases, the percentage inhibition rapidly increases not only for sparfloxacin but also for moxifloxacin and gatifloxacin (table 4) [8]. Pre-clinical data has recently become available that raises concern about the possibility of cardiovascular adverse events occurring when using these drugs, although at present there is no corresponding clinical data to match this. However, both moxifloxacin and sparfloxacin are recognised as causing corrected QT (QTc) interval prolongation, while this is not a problem associated with levofloxacin. Pre-clinical data available make a strong case for the safety of levofloxacin in comparison to other fluoroquinolones.

Another potential adverse event associated with fluoroquinolones is that of connective tissue disorders, and arthropathies [9]. Animal studies have shown an impact on tendons associated with administration of fluoroquinolones, and the effect appears to be sustained for several months. Achilles tendinitis has been investigated in association with fluoroquinolones, and it has been shown that compared to a reference of 1, the risk ratio of developing Achilles tendinitis is 10.1 with ofloxacin, and 2.8 for ciprofloxacin. Thus, the clinician needs to be aware of this potential problem, which is more likely to occur in patients also taking steroids.

Conclusion

The newer fluoroquinolones show sustained superiority over their older predecessors and may be considered preferred agents. With the development of these newer fluoroquinolones has come the need to differentiate among them based on their safety and tolerability profiles. It is now well recognised that levofloxacin has no QTc prolongation, a very low phototoxic potential, and does not interact with theophylline or warfarin. In contrast, sparfloxacin is associated with cardiac manifestations of QTc prolongation and has a high phototoxicity potential. Moxifloxacin is currently under observation with regard to QTc effects. The clarification of these differences allows the physician to prescribe fluoroquinolones, based not only upon their efficacy, but also their safety in individual patients.

References

1 Kim MK, Nightingale CH: Pharmacokinetics and pharmacodynamics of the fluoroquinolones; in Andriole VT (ed): The Quinolones, ed 3. San Diego, Academic Press, 2000, pp 169–202.
2 Lubasch A, Keller I, Borner K, Koeppe P, Lode H: Comparative pharmacokinetics of ciprofloxacin, gatifloxacin, grepafloxacin, levofloxacin, trovafloxacin, and moxifloxacin after single oral administration in healthy volunteers. Antimicrob Agents Chemother 2000;44:2600–2603.
3 Chien SC, Rogge MC, Gisclon LG, Curtin C, Wong F, Natarajan J, Williams RR, Fowler CL, Cheung WK, Chow AT: Pharmacokinetic profile of levofloxacin following once-daily 500-milligram oral or intravenous doses. Antimicrob Agents Chemother 1997;41:2256–2260.
4 Stahlmann R, Lode H: Safety overview: Toxicity, adverse effects, and drug interactions; in Andriole VT (ed): The Quinolones, ed 3. San Diego, Academic Press, 2000.
5 Höffken G, Borner K, Glatzel PD, Koeppe P, Lode H: Reduced enteral absorption of ciprofloxacin in the presence of antacids (letter). Eur J Clin Microbiol 1985;4:345.
6 Dembry LM, Farrington JM, Andriole VT: Fluoroquinolone antibiotics: Adverse effect and safety profiles. Infect Dis Clin Pract 1999;8:421–428.
7 Deppermann KM, Lode H: Fluoroquinolones: Interaction profile during enteral absorption. Drugs 1993;45(suppl 3):65–72.
8 Ball P, Mandell L, Niki Y, Tillotson G: Comparative tolerability of the newer fluoroquinolone antibacterials. Drug Saf 1999;21:407–421.
9 van der Linden PD, van de Lei J, Nab HW, Knol A, Stricker BH: Achilles tendinitis associated with fluoroquinolones. Br J Clin Pharmacol 1999;48:433–437.

Chemotherapy

Chemotherapy 2001;47(suppl 3):32–37

Latest Industry Information on the Safety Profile of Levofloxacin in the US

James B. Kahn

Infectious Disease Research, Ortho-McNeil Pharmaceutical Inc, Raritan, N.J., USA

Key Words

Fluoroquinolones · Levofloxacin · ADRs · Safety · PMS data · Toxicity · Clinical trials

Abstract

This paper reviews the safety data for levofloxacin utilizing reports from clinical and post-marketing surveillance trials. The side effect incidence rates are 1.3% for nausea, 0.1% for anxiety, 0.3% for insomnia, and 0.1% for headache. No levofloxacin-related adverse events were reported at a rate higher than 1.3%, and most were lower. Four clinical trials were reported. Levofloxacin achieved superior clinical and microbiological results compared to ceftriaxone/macrolide combination, and was better tolerated. Results comparing IV azithromycin plus ceftriaxone versus 500 mg levofloxacin in hospitalised CAP demonstrated that levofloxacin performed better, with more adverse events associated with the comparators (levofloxacin 5.3%, comparators 9.3%). High-dose levofloxacin (750 mg) was also evaluated and found to be well tolerated. Surveillance data reported low ADR rates for levofloxacin: nausea 0.8%, rash 0.5%, abdominal pain 0.4%, and diarrhoea, dizziness, and vomiting 0.3%. Worldwide and US surveillance data confirmed that tendon rupture occurred in less than 4 per million prescriptions, taste perversion in less than 3 per million, convulsions in 2 per million, and photosensitivity, hepatitis, hepatic failure, QT prolongation, torsade de pointes or empyema all in less than 1 per million.

Introduction

Levofloxacin, the first of the new fluoroquinolones approved for use in the US market, was launched in 1997. Since that time, it has been widely used for treating a range of

KARGER

Fax + 41 61 306 12 34
E-Mail karger@karger.ch
www.karger.com

0009–3157/01/0479–0032$17.50/0

Accessible online at:
www.karger.com/journals/che

James B. Kahn, MD
Infectious Disease Research
Ortho-McNeil Pharmaceutical Inc.
1000 Route 202, P.O. Box 300
Raritan, NJ 08869-0602 (USA)

infections, although its primary use remains in the respiratory setting. With proven efficacy based upon its excellent antibacterial spectrum, high penetration into sites of infection, and pharmacokinetic features, levofloxacin is sure to remain one of the most widely used fluoroquinolones available to the clinician. With an increasing array of other fluoroquinolones now becoming available, many with unacceptable adverse events, it is important to confirm the safety profiles of all agents. With this in mind, an all-encompassing review of the safety profile of levofloxacin in the US was prepared. This review builds upon all pre-launch data, adding the latest safety reports from clinical and post-marketing surveillance (PMS) sources.

Validity of Safety Data

When assessing safety data and reports of adverse events, it is important that the researcher be aware of all possible biases associated with the source of the data. In order to gain a wide understanding of the safety of an individual agent one most look at many different sources of data. This comprehensive update includes PMS data as well as results from four new clinical trials carried out in the US. Each of these methods of obtaining safety data has inherent biases. For example, post-marketing trials are vulnerable to disease effects, which are often reported as adverse events, but which are not related to the drug. This then gives an artificially high adverse drug reaction (ADR) rate. Results of safety analyses from randomised comparative trials are useful, but unfortunately, when assessing newer fluoroquinolones, there are few head-to-head studies evaluating their efficacy, let alone safety. Thus, reliable comparisons are difficult to make. Spontaneous reports from health care workers are seen as providing the best and broadest data, but this is highly dependent on temporal and secular factors. Data derived from the pharmaceutical company monitoring of levofloxacin is very conservative in nature. Thus, even if patients fall and hurt themselves while taking the drug, it may be reported as an adverse event, possibly related to dizziness, giving an unrealistically high ADR rate. Therefore, the advantages and disadvantages of the primary source need to be kept in mind when evaluating safety reports.

Levofloxacin — Updating the FDA Approved Package Insert

An update on the US safety data shows that there have been virtually no changes to the package insert since levofloxacin was first marketed. This package insert states that the side-effect incidence rates are highest for nausea at 1.3%. Central nervous system ADR rates are very low, 0.1% anxiety and 3% insomnia, and headache in 0.1%. In fact, no drug-related adverse events were reported at a rate higher than 1.3%, and the majority of side effects were even lower. The only two changes in the package insert are a note that there may be elevated prothrombin time when coadministered with warfarin, plus a modest new precaution about corrected QT interval (QTc) prolongation. This contrasts with the bolded warning required for other fluoroquinolones concerning potential cardiovascular effects, and is not class labelling. While many of the other new fluoroquinolones are now being found to be associated with prolongation of the QTc interval leading to subsequent cardiac events, this is only a very mild precaution with levofloxacin. None of the evidence to date indicates clinically relevant cardiac adverse events associated with levofloxacin usage. The warfarin warning was

Table 1. Levofloxacin safety profile (US clinical trial: n = 269)

Adverse drug reactions[a]	Levofloxacin (%)	Comparator (%)
Diarrhoea	4.5	7.3
Injection site pain	0.8	5.1
Infection site reaction	0	2.2
Insomnia	3.8	0.7
Moniliasis	0.8	2.9
Nausea	3.8	9.5

[a] Events with a difference of ≥2% between groups.

inserted following data derived from older patients who developed a higher incidence of warfarin-related bleeding. No clinical interaction has ever been noted, but there may be an elevated prothrombin time when levofloxacin and warfarin are administered at the same time.

Efficacy and Safety Data Derived from the Latest Clinical Trials

Four clinical trials have been performed in the US since 1997, which assess levofloxacin either alone or in comparison to other commonly used agents. The first of the clinical trials investigated 500 mg levofloxacin once daily versus intravenous ceftriaxone and erythromycin, changing to amoxicillin–clavulanic acid and clarithromycin in serious community-acquired pneumonia (CAP). This was defined as three or more American Thoracic Society (ATS) criteria for admission, plus mechanical ventilation or severe derangement of two or more vital signs. Illustrating that the patients selected for this trial comprised a very severe subgroup, the overall mortality rate was 9%. This study is very important as little data has been available in the past regarding the use of the fluoroquinolones in seriously ill patients, and in such situations they have generally been used in combination with other drugs. However, results from this trial make it clear that levofloxacin, used alone, was better than or as effective as the comparator arm.

Following antibiotic administration, levofloxacin achieved superior clinical and microbiological results than ceftriaxone and the macrolides. The clinical success with levofloxacin was 89%, and the microbiological eradication rate was 85%. In comparison, the combination therapy arm was only able to achieve an 84% clinical success rate and a 75% microbiological eradication rate.

Concerning ADRs, levofloxacin was better tolerated than the comparators. When all drug-related adverse events were analysed, there was a difference of at least 2% between the two groups. Levofloxacin ADR data were generally lower for insomnia, and the gastrointestinal side effects were predictably higher in the comparator arm. Diarrhoea, the most common side effect, occurred in 4.5% of levofloxacin-treated patients compared to a greater incidence of 7.3% in the comparator arm. Adverse events with a difference of greater than 2% between the two groups included diarrhoea, injection site pain, infection site reaction, insomnia, moniliasis, and nausea (table 1). Levofloxacin achieved superior microbiological results and had fewer ADRs when compared to ceftriaxone and the macrolides in this study.

Another study compared intravenous azithromycin plus ceftriaxone versus 500 mg levofloxacin in hospitalised patients with CAP. These patients were admitted with a Fine score between 70 and 130. Results from this trial confirmed that levofloxacin performed better, with a clinical success rate of

94%, compared to 92% for the comparator arm. The ADR rate was generally higher in the comparator arm, with an overall rate of 5.3% for levofloxacin compared to a much higher 9.3% for the alternative agents. Diarrhoea and vein disorders were not seen with levofloxacin, and dizziness was noted in only 0.9% (table 2). In sharp contrast, diarrhoea occurred in 4.2% of the comparators, vein disorders were reported at a rate of 2.5%, and pruritus occurred in 1.7%. Thus, levofloxacin again achieved superior clinical results and a better safety record than the comparator arm.

Results from a large open-label, non-comparative, surveillance trial of over 2000 patients, some with drug-resistant *S. pneumoniae*, revealed a clinical success rate of 95.3% for levofloxacin and a microbiological eradication rate of 94.7%. Using data from this large patient group, the most common adverse events all occurred at uniformly low rates. Nausea was seen in only 0.8%, rash in 0.5%, abdominal pain in 0.4%, and diarrhoea, dizziness, and vomiting in 0.3% (table 3).

The fourth clinical trial recently used levofloxacin in managing skin and soft tissue infections (SSTI). This compared levofloxacin 750 mg versus ticarcillin changing to amoxicillin–clavulanic acid. In this study, the higher dose of 750 mg of levofloxacin was used because the US Food and Drug Administration (FDA) defines complicated SSTI as generally having impaired vascularity. Thus, a dose higher than the usual 500 mg daily was used to ensure higher tissue concentrations. Trial results demonstrated a clinical success rate of 84% for levofloxacin compared to 80% for the other agents. The microbiological eradication rate associated with levofloxacin use was 87%, while the comparator arm only achieved a 74% eradication rate. In terms of safety, both arms of the study had a similar drug-related adverse event rate of 5%, showing that even at a higher dose, levofloxacin maintains excellent tolerability (table 4). In this study, when all adverse events were reported, including those that were not proven to be drug-related, levofloxacin had a rate of 46% compared to a higher 54% for the comparators. Of these, 10% were serious in the levofloxacin arm and 9% in the comparator arm. There were two deaths in both groups, although these were not shown to be related to the antibiotics, and there were no reports of unexpected adverse events occurring.

Table 2. Levofloxacin safety profile (US clinical trial: n = 269)

Adverse drug reactions[a]	Levofloxacin (%)	Comparator (%)
All body systems	5.3	9.3
Diarrhoea	0	4.2
Vein disorder	0	2.5
Pruritis	0	1.7
Dizziness	0.9	0
Insomnia	0.9	0

[a] Events with a difference of ≥2% between groups.

Table 3. Levofloxacin safety profile (US non-comparative clinical trial: n = 1,923)

Adverse drug reactions[a]	Incidence (%)
Nausea	0.8
Rash	0.5
Abdominal pain	0.4
Diarrhoea	0.3
Dizziness	0.3
Vomiting	0.3

[a] Events with a difference of ≥2% between groups.

Table 4. Adverse events in a study of 400 patients with skin and soft tissue infections

Adverse events	Levofloxacin	Comparator
All events	46%	54%
Serious events	10%	9%
Drug-related events	5%	5%
Deaths	2 patients	2 patients

Table 5. Reporting rates in the US of adverse drug reactions associated with levofloxacin

Reports of interest[a]	Reporting rate per million prescriptions
Tendon rupture	<4
Taste perversion	<3
Convulsions	2
Photosensitivity	<1
Hepatitis	<1
Hepatic failure	<1
QT prolongation	<1
Torsade de pointes	<1
Empyema[b]	<1

[a] Regardless of attribution.
[b] All organisms.

Spontaneous Report Rates of Adverse Events Associated with Levofloxacin

Spontaneous adverse events reported, regardless of attribution, also added weight to the safety of levofloxacin. These were compiled from data covering the 39-month period since the launch of levofloxacin in the US. They include any possible problem, even a rumor of such an event. All ADRs, including worldwide data and unlabelled ADRs, are then sent from the pharmaceutical company to the FDA. The reporting rate for adverse events associated with levofloxacin is then calculated using current prescription totals. Thus, the following data is total reporting rates, not an incidence rate based upon reporting rate assumptions. Data derived from more than 15 million prescriptions in the US, or 109 million prescriptions worldwide, demonstrated that tendon rupture occurred at a rate of less than 4 per million prescriptions, taste perversion in less than 3 per million, convulsions in only 2 per million, and photosensitivity, hepatitis, hepatic failure, QT prolongation, torsade de pointes, or empyema all occurred in less than 1 per million (table 5). These were all extremely low rates, and allowed the researchers to conclude that levofloxacin is a very safe antimicrobial worldwide.

Conclusions

The overall safety profile for levofloxacin remains as excellent as it was in 1997, with a reassuring lack of rare or unexpected events reported. It is particularly important to note that there have been no hints of any of the problems that have plagued other members of the fluoroquinolone class of antimicrobials. The issues of hepatotoxicity and cardiac effects that have marred some of the other newer fluoroquinolones do not appear to be an issue associated with administration of levofloxacin. This excellent safety record is upheld, even when the actual definition of safety is broadened to include reasonable reassurance of clinical efficacy and prolonged utility, continued excellent success rates, and a continued absence of emerging resistance of clinical significance.

Results of both clinical trials, phase IV trials, and spontaneous ADR reports are presented, showing that levofloxacin has not been associated with any significant phototoxicity, hepatic, cardiovascular, or other adverse events. Thus, the vast amount of safety data from these clinical trials, phase IV data and spontaneous reports will not have a significant impact on subsequent label revisions. The exceptional safety of levofloxacin has been confirmed by this recent US data and upheld by the PMS assessment of more than 130 million prescriptions of levofloxacin worldwide.

Chemotherapy

Chemotherapy 2001;47(suppl 3):38–43

Latest Industry Information on the Safety Profile of Levofloxacin in Japan

Katsuro Yagawa

Drug Safety Administration Department, Daiichi Pharmaceutical Co., Ltd., Tokyo, Japan

Key Words

Levofloxacin · Fluoroquinolones · Adverse drug reaction · Safety · Post-marketing surveillance data · Toxicity

Abstract

This paper focuses on the development of four major adverse drug reactions (ADRs) associated with some fluoroquinolones: convulsions, phototoxicity, cardiac effects, and hepatotoxicity. CNS adverse events have been linked to fluoroquinolone administration, including seizures, which are more likely with co-administration of NSAIDs. Only 61 cases of convulsions have been reported with levofloxacin, with 33 of those affected having received NSAIDs. The assumed rate of serious convulsions was as low as 1/65,000 with NSAIDs and 1/260,000 without NSAIDs. Levofloxacin has a very low phototoxicity-inducing potential confirmed by pre-clinical animal studies and the results of post-marketing surveillance (PMS). Pre-clinical results demonstrated that levofloxacin was 20 times less phototoxic than sparfloxacin and PMS data show that serious phototoxicity develops in only 1 in 1.8 million cases treated with levofloxacin. While many fluoroquinolones are associated with cardiac effects, pre-clinical data has shown that compared with sparfloxacin and grepafloxacin, levofloxacin has no effect on myocardial conduction. PMS data further support the safety of levofloxacin in this regard. While trovafloxacin is associated with serious hepatic problems, PMS data demonstrates that levofloxacin has a very low incidence of 1/100,000 hepatic effects. These results were confirmed in a prospective study that confirmed a low 1.3% incidence rate for all ADRs associated with levofloxacin.

Introduction

Levofloxacin, the *l*-isomer of ofloxacin, was launched in Japan in 1993. As the first country in which levofloxacin was marketed,

KARGER

Fax + 41 61 306 12 34
E-Mail karger@karger.ch
www.karger.com

0009–3157/01/0479–0038$17.50/0

Accessible online at:
www.karger.com/journals/che

Katsuro Yagawa
Daiichi Pharmaceutical Co., Ltd.
14-10 Nihonbashi
3-chome, Chuo-ku
Tokyo, Japan 103-8234

Table 1. Serious adverse drug reactions caused by some new fluoroquinolones

Year	New quinolones	Serious ADRs	Period between launch and occurrence of problem
1985	Enoxacin	Seizure (interaction with NSAIDs)	6 months
1992	Temafloxacin	Haemolytic anaemia Hypoglycaemia	10 months
1995	Sparfloxacin	Photodermatosis QT prolongation	8 months (in France)
1998	Trovafloxacin	Serious hepatic reactions Pancreatitis	5 months
1999	Trovafloxacin	Serious hepatic reactions	16 months
1999	Grepafloxacin	Severe cardiovascular events	about 2 years

Japan has developed an extensive database of information on this agent, providing important safety statistics. Since its initial introduction, use of levofloxacin has grown rapidly, with more than 90 million Japanese patients treated with this agent. With another 40 million treated worldwide, there is now data from over 130 million prescriptions globally. This huge, comprehensive database provides extremely valuable information on any possible, as well as any unexpected, adverse events that may have arisen. Such a large pool of patients treated means that the statistics available are extremely reliable, and provide information on the use of levofloxacin across many age groups, racial and ethnic categories, as well as other selected patient populations. The importance of having such extensive safety data cannot be emphasized too strongly, as many of the newer fluoroquinolones have fallen into disrepute following the development of unexpected and unacceptable side effects.

Serious adverse drug reactions (ADRs) caused by some new quinolones have been reported since 1985. The time from launching the agent until recognition of side effects differed among the individual fluoroquinolones. Often the side effects developed within quite a short time frame from launch of the drug into the market place, ranging from 5 months to 2 years (table 1). For example, the serious hepatic reactions associated with trovafloxacin were recognised within 5 months of its introduction into the market, and within 16 months, reported reactions were severe enough to lead to its withdrawal. Other agents that have been introduced, only to have severe reactions associated with their use, include enoxacin, temafloxacin, sparfloxacin, and grepafloxacin. With this in mind, it is important to note that levofloxacin has been used for over 6 years in Japan and results from a large post-marketing surveillance (PMS) study confirm the continuing safety of this agent. This paper focuses on the development of four major ADRs associated with some fluoroquinolones: convulsions, especially when administered at the same time as non-steroidal anti-inflammatory drugs (NSAIDs), phototoxicity, cardiac effects, and hepatotoxicity. These are now thought to be common to virtually all of the new fluoroquinolones to various degrees, constituting a class effect.

Table 2. Incidence of clonic convulsions related to levofloxacin, in patients taking and not taking NSAIDs from 6-year post-marketing surveillance data in Japan

Patient receiving NSAIDs	All adverse events		Serious adverse events	
	cases	incidence[a]	cases	incidence[a]
Yes	33	1/53,000	27	1/65,000
No	28	1/250,000	27	1/260,000

[a] 10% assumed event-reporting date.

Central Nervous System — Seizures Associated with Fluoroquinolones

A range of central nervous system (CNS) adverse events have been linked to fluoroquinolone administration, including the development of seizures. The induction of convulsions by fluoroquinolones can occur when the drug is administered alone, or can be dramatically increased in both incidence and severity during concomitant administration of NSAIDs. This is illustrated by enoxacin. In 1985, within 6 months of being launched, it was reported that enoxacin was associated with seizures. Investigation of this early fluoroquinolone had indicated that it had a low convulsion-inducing activity when used alone. However, this was found to increase by a factor of more than 800 when used with 4-biphenyl acetic acid, the active metabolite of fenbufen, one of the commonly used NSAIDs. In contrast, the likelihood of levofloxacin inducing a convulsion only increases minimally when used at the same time as NSAIDs. The data from the 6-year PMS period confirmed the safety of levofloxacin in this regard. During this time, only 61 cases of convulsions were reported, and 33 of these had received concomitant NSAID therapy (table 2). Assuming a 10% reporting rate, the incidence of convulsions, when levofloxacin was used with NSAIDs, was 1/53,000, and when used alone, 1/250,000, a 5-fold difference. These results highlight the relative safety of levofloxacin, which appears to be less likely to cause seizures than other fluoroquinolones.

Phototoxicity — A Serious Problem for Sparfloxacin

It has been reported that phototoxicity is a class effect associated with new quinolones. However, there is now compelling data showing that levofloxacin has a very low phototoxicity-inducing potential. This data was derived from both preclinical animal studies as well as PMS study IV. In the preclinical studies, a number of fluoroquinolones, including levofloxacin and sparfloxacin, were orally administered to mice. The mice were then irradiated with ultraviolet light for 4 h, and the thickness of their auricular skin was measured at 24 h. The dosage required to induce a 50% thickening in skin was then calculated. Results from this study demonstrated that levofloxacin was 20 times less phototoxic than sparfloxacin.

Clinical data has since become available which also supports the safety of levofloxacin in this regard. Only 45 cases of levofloxacin-induced phototoxicity have been reported in the 6-year PMS study, yielding an estimated incidence of 1/200,000, assuming a 10% event-reporting rate (table 3). Adding even more weight to the safety of levofloxacin is the

Table 3. Incidence of photodermatosis from six-year post-marketing surveillance data in Japan

	All cases of photosensitivity		Serious cases	
	cases	incidence	cases	incidence
Sparfloxacin[a]	53	1/189	–	–
Levofloxacin	45	1/200,000[b]	5	1/1,760,000[b]

[a] Data from package insert in Japan.
[b] 10% assumed event-reporting-rate.

fact that of these, only 5 were classified as serious, giving a very low incidence of 1/1.8 million. In contrast, sparfloxacin induced a higher incidence of phototoxic reactions. When this latter fluoroquinolone was used, 1/189 cases developed phototoxic side effects. In France, these problems with sparfloxacin were recognized in 1995, within 8 months of sparfloxacin's introduction. This significant problem for sparfloxacin greatly inhibits its usefulness. In comparison, levofloxacin appears to have a very low phototoxic potential with minimal clinical impact.

Cardiac Effects Associated with Fluoroquinolones

Myocardial conduction disturbance is a potentially serious adverse event associated with new quinolones that has recently attracted attention. The first indication that fluoroquinolones may cause this problem was reported in 1995, when it was shown that patients taking sparfloxacin developed corrected QT interval (QTc) prolongation. Since that time, this adverse event has been reported for a number of other fluoroquinolones, leading to the general belief that this is a class effect associated with all of these agents. However, as data that is more comprehensive has become available, it has become apparent that while many of the fluoroquinolones are responsible for this, levofloxacin is an exceptional agent, which can be described as virtually free of myocardial effects. Recent data has shown that compared with sparfloxacin and grepafloxacin, levofloxacin has no effect on myocardial conduction in vitro (unpublished data). Statistics from the PMS study reveal that worldwide there have only been 8 cases of QTc prolongation or torsade de pointes associated with levofloxacin, giving an incidence of 1/1.6 million (assuming a 10% event-reporting rate). When the Japanese data is looked at individually, only 1 case of cardiac effects was reported, giving rise to an incredibly low rate of 1/8.8 million (table 4). This data is exceptional because there have been such a large number of levofloxacin prescriptions made throughout the world, with very careful monitoring. Thus, the cardiac safety of this agent seems assured. In contrast, the package inserts as requested by the US

Table 4. Incidence of torsade de pointes associated with levofloxacin from 6-year post-marketing surveillance data in Japan

	Cases	Incidence[a]
Worldwide	8	1/1.6 million
Japan	1	1/8.8 million

[a] 10% assumed event-reporting-rate.

Table 5. Incidence of serious hepatic adverse reactions

	Estimated sum of prescriptions	Serious hepatic ADR	Incidence of serious hepatic ADR
Trovafloxacin [a] (worldwide)	2.5 million (launch May 1999)	140	1/1,800
Levofloxacin (Japan)	88 million (launch September 1999)	87	1/100,000[b]
Levofloxacin (worldwide)	125 million (launch September 1999)	115	1/109,000[b]

[a] Data from press release by US FDA and UK MCA.
[b] 10% assumed event-reporting-rate.

Food and Drug Administration (FDA) in the US for moxifloxacin and gatifloxacin warn about the possibility of myocardial conduction disturbances, while levofloxacin only has this noted as a possible class effect.

Hepatic Adverse Effects — A Significant Problem for Trovafloxacin Leading to Its Withdrawal

Trovafloxacin, a new fluoroquinolone, was prescribed to 2.5 million patients worldwide from its launch until May 1999. During this short period, 140 cases of serious hepatic failure, including 9 cases of death or hepatic transplantation were reported. Trovafloxacin is associated with serious hepatic events in 1/1,800 subjects (table 5). This data was reported to the FDA, and due to the serious nature of this problem, trovafloxacin was in effect withdrawn from the market. Concern has arisen regarding the potential of other fluoroquinolones to also cause hepatic problems. However, figures from the levofloxacin PMS trial demonstrate that, in Japan, levofloxacin has been prescribed to 88 million subjects with only 87 patients reporting serious hepatic problems, yielding a very low incidence of 1/100,000. Worldwide data confirms this, with an even lower incidence globally of 1/109,000.

As well as the adverse event of hepatic failure, there have been recent studies into the cytotoxicity of fluoroquinolones. Comparative data on the toxicity of various new quinolones against hepatoblastoma (Hep G2) cells has demonstrated the safety of levofloxacin compared to other fluoroquinolones. Trovafloxacin was cytotoxic at a concentration of less than 1 μg/ml, whereas levofloxacin, even at a 20-fold higher concentration, was virtually without cytotoxicity. Although the in vitro data does not necessarily indicate hepatopathy in human subjects, these results also add to the clinical results, which indicate that the risk of hepatotoxicity with levofloxacin is very low.

When adverse events other than the four main types discussed above were analysed, 702 cases of serious ADRs were found for which a causal relationship with levofloxacin could not be ruled out during the 6-year PMS trial. This covered all possible reactions, resulting in a very low adverse event rate.

Prospective Safety Evaluation — A 1.3% Incidence of ADRs for Levofloxacin

While the PMS data is extremely comprehensive for levofloxacin, there is additional evidence supporting its safety and tolerability. The occurrence of ADRs was also prospectively investigated in 33,000 cases, each treated with either levofloxacin or ofloxacin. Ofloxacin, the parent compound of levofloxacin, has been used for a very long time, and it remains one of the safest fluoroquinolones. Results from this prospective study confirmed a 1.3% incidence rate for all ADRs associated with levofloxacin, and a 2.6% incidence rate with ofloxacin (fig. 1). Ofloxacin has been the most widely used fluoroquinolone worldwide over the past 15 years, administered to more than 300 million people. Therefore, levofloxacin has been proven to be quite a bit safer than its parent compound, ofloxacin, which has been considered a model of safety.

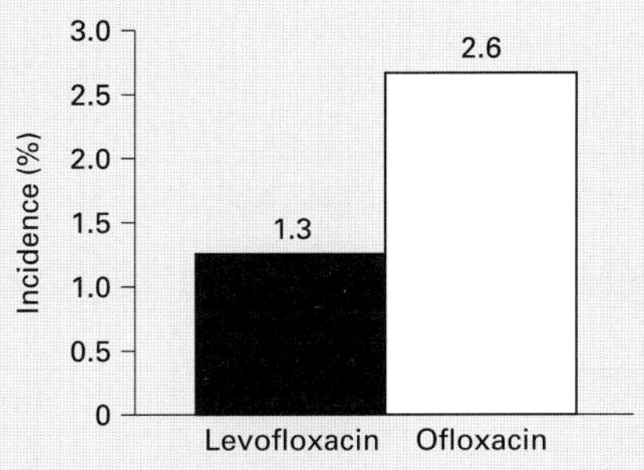

Fig. 1. Comparison of the incidence of adverse drug reactions in Japan.

Conclusion

Levofloxacin was first launched in Japan in 1993, and has since been prescribed to more than 90 million Japanese patients. Investigations presented include stringent 6-year PMS results and prospective study findings. During this study period, levofloxacin has had virtually no reports of cardiac adverse events. Since its introduction, the incidence of CNS adverse events in patients treated with levofloxacin has been very low, and this remains low even when levofloxacin is taken in combination with NSAIDs. Phototoxicity is recognized as a class effect associated with the new fluoroquinolones. However, the incidence of this problem with levofloxacin is very low, although not non-existent. The rate of hepatic adverse events was also very low, and prospective study results confirm that levofloxacin is equivalent to, or better than, ofloxacin in terms of safety. Clinicians can continue to use levofloxacin, confident of its excellent safety record.

Chemotherapy

Chemotherapy 2001;47(suppl 3):44–46

General Discussion

Following the presentations, a thought-provoking discussion took place between all faculty members and the audience. The major issues of concern to physicians working with fluoroquinolones were debated, including safety data and optimal administration schedules. The consensus of the discussion was that levofloxacin is a very well tolerated agent, even when used at high doses and for a long duration. Cross-resistance among the fluoroquinolones is a potential problem, but the degree to which this occurs varies among individual agents. To overcome the development of resistance, it may be best to use a high dose, once daily. This administration schedule is possible with levofloxacin. The following report outlines the most important issues raised during this session.

Questioner: What is the longest duration of therapy using levofloxacin for which you have safety data?

Dr. Kahn: We have results from a trial conducted in the US that investigated a once-daily 500-mg dose, orally administered to patients with osteomyelitis. Due to the chronic nature of the infection, some of the patients in this study were treated for periods of up to six months. Data from approximately 100 patients treated for this long duration revealed no difference in their side-effect profile, compared to patients treated with a shorter duration of levofloxacin. We also have anecdotal evidence arising from the use of levofloxacin in tuberculosis. Levofloxacin is recommended as a preferred agent in treating multidrug-resistant tuberculosis (MDR-TB). In these cases, levofloxacin is used at a high dose of 750 mg or 1,000 mg, once daily, for several months. It appears to be safe and well tolerated in these situations. Ofloxacin, the parent compound of levofloxacin, has been used for many years in MDR-TB strategies, where a long duration of therapy is utilised. In this situation, it appears to be very well tolerated.

Questioner: Is it possible to extrapolate results from ofloxacin, and to state that since ofloxacin is safe both under normal use and for longer duration, that levofloxacin will also be safe following long periods of administration?

Dr. Kahn: In theory, this appears to be true. As the parent compound, the safety of ofloxacin will extend to ensuring the safety of levofloxacin. We know that ofloxacin contains the two rotatory isomers, both dextro- and levo-forms. Levofloxacin only contains the levo-

KARGER

Fax + 41 61 306 12 34
E-Mail karger@karger.ch
www.karger.com

0009–3157/01/0479–0044$17.50/0

Accessible online at:
www.karger.com/journals/che

isomer. What is not known is whether the dextrorotatory isomer, which ofloxacin contains, is protective. This cannot be ruled out. Therefore, to confirm the safety of levofloxacin when used for a long duration, we need prolonged surveillance results.

Dr. Lode: Dr. Kahn, do you have toxicological data for six-month administration schedules, and did you need this for FDA approval?

Dr. Kahn: We have toxicological data for three-month administration of levofloxacin and have approval to treat for this length of time. However, the FDA has very rigid requirements, which only allow humans to be treated for a long duration after murine models have been used for the same duration. Thus, we do not have toxicological data for six-month administration.

Dr. Rubinstein: Dr. Yagawa, do you have any data on the long-term use of levofloxacin in animals?

Dr. Yagawa: We do not have data from animal studies investigating long-term use of levofloxacin. However, we do have anecdotal evidence following its use in patients with leprosy. A problem with this is that it only includes a small number of patients, making it hard to draw firm conclusions about toxicity. In Japan, many patients have been treated with levofloxacin or ofloxacin for tuberculosis, using long-term treatment schedules. However, we do not have enough data to provide firm toxicological long-term data supporting the safety of levofloxacin in this situation, although it appears to be well tolerated by the majority of patients.

Questioner: Is there any data available regarding the incidence of side effects associated with levofloxacin among different races?

Dr. Yagawa: Racial differences in incidence of adverse drug-events have not been looked at closely. It is difficult to assess racial differences between Asians and Europeans in terms of levofloxacin safety, because a different dose is often used in Asians (300 mg) compared to Europeans (500 mg). Any differences that may appear could be related to changes in body size, with smaller Asians potentially more at risk of developing side effects if they use the European dose.

Dr. Kahn: Over the past few years, the FDA has encouraged us to collect race-specific data. However, we do not have that data at present, and when it is incorporated into future trials, it will probably only look at differences between black and white patients. Thus, it will be difficult to make clear comparisons between Asians and Europeans in terms of the tolerability of levofloxacin. I think that a larger concern is ensuring that the individual patient receives the appropriate dose. For instance, a large Asian person treated with a 300-mg dose may not be receiving the best administration schedule. We need to resolve questions related to dose based on the size of the patient and real-world kinetics. It may be that we need more choices of available doses.

Questioner: What is the maximum safe dosage of levofloxacin?

Dr. Kahn: Safety data has been compiled for 1,000-mg doses in normal volunteers, where the peak concentration (C_{max}) following a single oral dose was 12 μg/ml, and the area under the plasma concentration-time curve (AUC) was vast.

Dr. Rubinstein: There is a need for more data outlining pharmacokinetics. The trend in the future will be to shorten the duration of therapy and increase the dose to get an initial maximal kill, in order to overcome the risk of selection for resistance. Thus, it is important that we obtain more specific information on the absolute safety and tolerability of higher doses among different-sized patients.

Questioner: What is the effect of the fluoroquinolone metabolites in the development of side effects?

Dr. Lode: At present, the effect of individual metabolites is not clear, although it does appear likely that those compounds which undergo less metabolisation, such as levofloxacin, may be associated with fewer side effects.

Questioner: Resistance to ciprofloxacin has become more apparent since its introduction. Is there any cross-resistance between ciprofloxacin-resistant isolates and resistance to other fluoroquinolones?

Dr. Acar: There is no question that there is cross-resistance among the fluoroquinolones, but in light of the latest research, this concept has to be modulated. It has now become apparent that cross-resistance is not equal among all of the members of this class. This is because of the different mechanisms operating behind the development of resistance, such as alterations in effects on DNA gyrase and topoisomerases, all of which may be affected to varying degrees. This is particularly true of the efflux system. Since the individual fluoroquinolones require different steps to occur before resistance develops, the degree of cross-resistance can fluctuate among these agents. Illustrating this is data that has shown that cross-resistance among the fluoroquinolones to *Staphylococcus aureus (S. aureus)* is not equal. While there are a number of methicillin-resistant *S. aureus* (MRSA) isolates that are highly resistant to ciprofloxacin, this does not mean that there is 100% resistance to all of the other fluoroquinolones. This is because some of the new fluoroquinolones have a lower minimum inhibitory concentration (MIC), and remain effective against some isolates that are resistant to less effective fluoroquinolones.

Questioner: Which administration schedule is more likely to result in the development of resistance — a once-daily or twice-daily schedule?

Dr. Rubinstein: From a basic scientific viewpoint, it is important to eradicate the organism as soon as possible, which is achieved by the highest dose that can be tolerated. Fluoroquinolone killing of bacteria is concentration dependent and extremely rapid. Since the bactericidal activity of all fluoroquinolones relates to the AUC, the highest dose tolerated would result in improved rates of bacterial kill. This would then translate into less re-growth, with a reduced chance of resistant mutants surviving. Therefore, on a theoretical basis, the initial dose should be increased to achieve maximal kill. If this is done, it may be possible to shorten the duration of treatment, which is an important area for future research. Thus, from a scientific rationale, a higher-dose, once-daily schedule would be less likely to result in resistance than a lower-dose, twice-daily schedule.

Chemotherapy

Chemotherapy 2001;47(suppl 3):47–48

Summary

Ethan Rubinstein, Symposium Chairperson

Department of Internal Medicine and Unit of Infectious Diseases, Tel Aviv University School of Medicine, Tel Aviv, Israel

Providing a base upon which the other presentations could build, I reviewed the historical development of fluoroquinolones, and then analysed the structure of individual agents in terms of their efficacy and tolerability, allowing the agents to be categorised based upon the likelihood of their causing adverse events due to their structure. This was followed by Professor Claude Carbon, who reported on differences between individual fluoroquinolones that have been described following use in patients. Such data is imperative in clearly defining which agents are safe to use, and highlight the fact that there are major differences now recognised. A number of agents have been withdrawn, such as trovafloxacin, and most recently, clinafloxacin. Of the agents remaining, levofloxacin appears to be extremely safe with a low rate of adverse events, and low rates of cardiac and hepatic problems. Professor Jacques F. Acar widened the discussion by comparing fluoroquinolones to other commonly used agents, such as macrolides and β-lactams. It is important to have a clear understanding of the side-effect profiles associated with all major classes of antimicrobials, and Professor Acar provided this. He then discussed one of the newer issues gaining importance in the infectious disease community — namely, the ecological impact of antimicrobials upon the normal human gastrointestinal flora. Levofloxacin was shown to have less of an impact on gastrointestinal flora than many other compounds, and was not associated with overgrowth of resistant mutants, unlike other agents. Professor Hartmut Lode discussed pharmacological differences among the fluoroquinolones. He drew attention to the many advantages possessed by the newer fluoroquinolones, such as levofloxacin. They maintain excellent pharmacokinetic profiles, making them easy and effective to use.

Actual clinical data following extensive use of levofloxacin was then used to assess its safety profile and compare it to the clinical adverse-event profiles for the other agents. This was first assessed from a US perspective, with results reported by Dr. James B. Kahn, followed by Japanese and global data reported by Dr. Katsuro Yagawa. They showed that even following six years of levofloxacin use,

KARGER

Fax + 41 61 306 12 34
E-Mail karger@karger.ch
www.karger.com

0009–3157/01/0479–0047$17.50/0

Accessible online at:
www.karger.com/journals/che

Ethan Rubinstein, MD
Department of Internal Medicine and Unit of Infectious Diseases
Chaim Sheba Medical Center, Tel Aviv University School of Medicine
Tel-Hashomer, 52621 (Israel)
Tel. +972 3 530350, Fax +972 3 5347081, E-Mail unit@netvision.net.il

the incidence of adverse events with this drug remains extremely low, with 1.3% of adverse events reported in Japan.

Following the presentations, there was a lively discussion focusing upon some of the most clinically important differences. The discussion allowed faculty and participants to join in a relaxed and stimulating environment to discuss and answer questions and issues related to the safety of fluoroquinolones. Participants attending from around the world took the opportunity to ask the distinguished panel their opinion on a range of important issues related to the safety of the fluoroquinolones. Throughout the roundtable discussion, it was apparent that levofloxacin is one of the most clinically effective fluoroquinolones, which is coupled with an extremely good safety profile.